DATE DUE

	DEC 1 4 2011	

Text Atlas of Wound Management

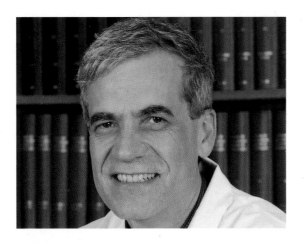

Vincent Falanga MD.
Dr Falanga is Professor of Dermatology at Boston University School of Medicine and Chairman of its Department of Dermatology at the Roger Williams Medical Center. A graduate of Harvard Medical School, he is board certified in dermatology and internal medicine. He is a fellow of the American College of Physicians. His main interests are chronic wounds, growth factors and bioengineered skin, and the basic science aspects of wound healing and fibrosis. He is the author of over 250 peer-reviewed articles and textbook chapters and co-author of '*Leg and Foot Ulcers: A Clinician's Guide*'. He is Section Editor for Wound Care for the *Journal of Dermatological Treatment*.

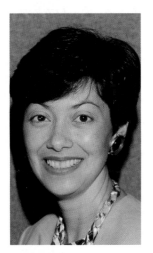

Tania J Phillips MD.
Dr Phillips is Professor of Dermatology at Boston University School of Medicine and a graduate of Guy's Hospital Medical School, University of London. She is a member of the Royal College of Physicians. Her research interests have focused on chronic wounds and the use of cultured skin and skin substitutes. She is also interested in skin problems in the elderly and in the assessment of quality of life in patients with chronic wounds. She is the author of over 100 publications and has co-authored three books.

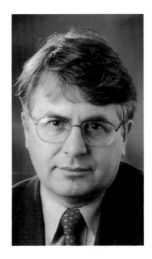

Keith G Harding MBChB.
Dr Harding graduated in medicine from the University of Birmingham in 1976. He is a member of the Royal College of General Practitioners and a Fellow of the Royal College of Surgeons and currently directs the Wound Healing Research Unit at the University of Wales College of Medicine and is Professor of Rehabilitation Medicine (Wound Healing). His main interests are in research, educational and service aspects of wound healing. He is the author of over 100 publications and is co-editor of *Wounds: Biology and Management* in addition to developing new journals and societies focused in the area of wound healing.

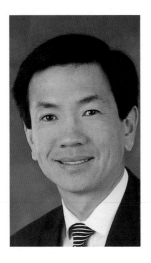

Ronald Moy MD.
Dr Moy graduated from Albany Medical College. He is an Associate Clinical Professor of Dermatology at the VA-West Los Angeles Medical Center, Chief of Dermatologic Surgery and a fellow of the American College of Mohs Micrographic Surgery. He is the author of over 100 publications and has co-authored four other books and is the Editor-in-Chief of *Dermatologic Surgery*. He is also in private practice specializing in cosmetic dermatologic surgery and skin cancer treatment.

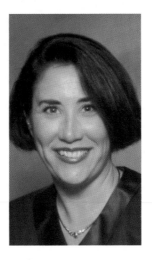

Lisa Peerson RN DNC.
A graduate of the Nursing School at Tulsa University in Oklahoma, she has spent most of her professional career in Miami, Florida. She began as a surgical nurse and then nurse manager at Cedars Medical Center. For the last 12 years she has been a nurse in the Department of Dermatology at the University of Miami. Her expertise is in skin and wound care and in the management of complex situations involving difficult to heal wounds.

Text Atlas of Wound Management

Edited by

Vincent Falanga MD FACP
Professor of Dermatology, Boston University School of Medicine and Chairman of Dermatology and Cutaneous Surgery at the Roger Williams Medical Center, Providence, Rhode Island, USA

with

Tania J Phillips MD
Professor of Dermatology, Boston University School of Medicine, Boston, Massachusetts, USA

Keith G Harding MBChB MRCGP FRCS
Professor of Rehabilitation Medicine (Wound Healing) and Director of the Wound Healing Unit, University of Wales College of Medicine, Cardiff, UK

Ronald Moy MD
Associate Clinical Professor, UCLA Division of Dermatology and Chief of Dermatologic Surgery, VA-WCH LA Medical Center, Los Angeles, California, USA

Lisa J Peerson RN DNC
Department of Dermatology and Cutaneous Surgery, University of Miami School of Medicine, Miami, Florida, USA

MARTIN DUNITZ

© Martin Dunitz Ltd 2000

First published in the United Kingdom in 2000 by

Martin Dunitz Ltd
The Livery House
7–9 Pratt Street
London NW1 0AE

A CIP record for this book is available from the British Library.

ISBN 1 85317 471 8

Distributed in the United States by:
Blackwell Science Inc.
Commerce Place, 350 Main Street
Malden, MA 02148, USA
Tel: 1-800-215-1000

Dsitributed in Canada by:
Login Brothers Book Company
324 Salteaux Crescent
Winnipeg, Manitoba, R3J 3T2
Canada
Tel: 204-224-4068

Distributed in Brazil by:
Ernesto Reichmann Distribuidora de Livros, Ltda
Rua Coronel Marques 335, Tatuape 03440-000
Sao Paulo
Brazil

Composition by Scribe Design, Gillingham, Kent
Printed and bound in Italy by Printer Trento Srl

Contents

Introduction

This is a pictorial guide to wound management. In preparing it, we had a rather broad audience in mind. The guide should prove useful to clinicians starting out and wanting to know more about wounds and how to care for them, to students, and to other professionals who need to have a pictorial reference and a working knowledge about this field. We also hope that this work will be of value to established clinicians who are already familiar with wounds and their management; it is often worthwhile to "compare notes" and find areas of agreement and disagreement. Out intent has been to keep and project an open mind about wound management. There is no doubt that in the next few years we will see an increased use of specific guidelines for how to deal with certain common wounds, e.g. venous, diabetic and pressure ulcers. However, a good number of the situations described in this guide fall outside definite diagnostic categories, or are complicated by other systemic or wound-related factors. Some conditions are simply uncommon or rare and do not allow a uniformly accepted management. Caring for patients with these conditions can be very challenging and requires a more pragmatic approach.

In preparing this pictorial guide, we established a number of goals. We wanted to provide readers with a broad exposure to cutaneous wounds, both acute and chronic. This overall goal became possible because of the variety of experiences of each contributor. In our opinion, it was also important that each photograph and the accompanying text be packaged in a clinical vignette which could stand on its own, without the reader having to refer back and forth to different portions of the guide. We think we have achieved this goal, albeit at the small cost of some repetitive remarks. Another essential goal was to provide our audience with a stimulating mix of purely clinical information and comments about the pathogenesis of the various conditions being discussed. This combined approach should be evident both in the rather extensive legends to each photograph and in the introduction to each section. We certainly do not claim that this pictorial management guide will take the place of more exhaustive works and textbooks on the science of wound healing, the pathogenic steps responsible for failure to heal, and wound dressings. In this regard, we hope that the selective bibliography will be helpful to those seeking additional information.

Yet another goal was to make the readers feel as though they were with us at the bedside or in the clinic, facing the same problems and challenges that we were dealing with. We hope that the rather informal, narrative approach we have adopted will serve that purpose. The clinical situations we have presented do not fall into the category of "show and tell". Rather, we hope that we have shown and projected our struggle in managing some difficult wounds. The management of some wounds remains uncharted territory, and there is often no absolutely right answer for their management; much depends not just on the condition being treated but on the patient's circumstances and environment.

The guide is divided into eight sections. The first is about wounds and ulcers due mainly to non-surgical injury. This section does not deal with "major" trauma, such as burns and other catastrophic events, which are best dealt with by surgeons who specialize in those areas. The second section addresses wounds created by scalpel, lasers, and other common office-based procedures. There is a certain amount of overlap between the first and second sections, which proved to be inevitable. Infection is the subject of the third section. There we deal with primary infections, which may cause the wound in the first place, as well as colonization and infection of existing wounds. Wounds due to pressure, such as diabetic ulcers, are the main topic of the fourth section. The reader may notice that we had some trouble separating purely vascular ulcers from wounds caused by inflammatory processes (fifth and sixth sections, respectively). We think that this difficulty simply reflects the reality of clinical practice. Indeed, we have noticed that clinicians well versed in the management of purely vascular wounds may have trouble at times dealing with inflammatory components which complicate their management. We actually hope that the degree of overlap we have provided in those two sections will be useful.

Neoplasms are not an extremely common cause of ulcers, at least in countries where there is good access to medical care. Still, tumors do ulcerate and, occasionally, present as ulcers; these are dealt with in section 7. Finally, in section 8, we have brought together certain practical points which are more general in nature and may be applicable to a variety of clinical situations. It is not that the other sections are not "practical". Indeed, the thrust of this guide is to provide a hands-on approach to diagnosis and wound management. However, we believe that it has been useful to use this last section as a way to condense our experience with dressings and to suggest ways to overcome unusual aspects of wound care.

We do hope that we have achieved at least some of our goals and that this work will ultimately help patients suffering from cutaneous wounds. The guide may be regarded as a starting point on how to think about managing a broad variety of wounds, and how to base the diagnostic and therapeutic approach on available evidence and still have the flexibility to adapt to the circumstances each patient presents.

Vincent Falanga

1 Acute wounds: response to injury

Introduction

In this section we have described some of the problems one deals with in the management of wounds caused by skin trauma or created by means other than scalpel surgery. The situations we have presented are common, and we hope that they provide the reader with reference points about how to manage some of these problems.

A fundamental difference of acute wounds not caused by the scalpel is their propensity for hyperpigmentation and hypopigmentation. In general, patients with darker skin are more susceptible to these complications and this fact has to be kept in mind when discussing treatment options and possible side-effects. Simple measures can often affect outcome in a very favorable way. For example, pretreatment with bleaching agents is thought to decrease the incidence of hyperpigmentation after trichloroacetic acid (TCA) peels. Simple skin care after TCA peels can also consist of the use of moisturizers and low-potency topical steroids. Healing is usually not a problem after TCA peels, but pretreatment with retinoic acid seems to accelerate resurfacing, and this approach has been used in other situations (e.g. with dermabrasion). It remains important to warn patients about the side-effects of these types of injuries and about the clinical course. For instance, hyperpigmentation is commonly transient and excessive redness tends to disappear within weeks.

Postoperative pain also seems to be more prevalent after these procedures (e.g. laser treatment) compared to scalpel-induced injury. We do not know the reasons for this, but it might be that damage is more diffuse and not confined or limited to the target area. Topical anesthesia with EMLA can be very useful in some circumstances. Postoperative dressings, especially occlusive dressings, can also improve the pain in a very dramatic fashion. Another advantage of occlusive dressings in these types of wounds is that they can control exudate and can lead to remarkable decreases in the amount of crusting and even scarring. In our opinion, the beneficial effects of occlusion on postoperative scarring have not been fully realized by many clinicians. How this comes about is not known. However, we do know that occlusion can decrease the inflammatory infiltrate, which can probably downregulate the deposition of extracellular matrix proteins and even decrease pain. The decrease in erythema seen with occlusive dressings after laser resurfacing is probably due to decreased inflammation, but a direct effect on vascular structures and nerve fibers cannot be excluded.

This section presents some common approaches to dressing wounds created by lasers, or TCA peels, or dermabrasion. These suggestions are what the authors have found useful and, indeed, similar approaches seem to be used by many clinicians. Foam and gel dressings are commonly used after laser surgery, for example. Some approaches are still quite experimental but are promising. For instance, the use of bioengineered skin after cosmetic surgery with lasers or dermabrasion is a very attractive notion. With these procedures, we are basically removing layers of skin (and cellular components) which have been damaged by sun exposure. It is very tantalizing to think that the addition of fresh young cells from bioengineered skin products could have a more permanent effect on the cosmetic outcome. The cells in bioengineered skin, which generally come from a neonatal source, are quite active from the proliferative and synthetic standpoint and, even if they do not remain in the recipient, are probably able to modify the healing response in a beneficial way.

A special clinical situation is that of wounds caused by the patient, either intentionally to gain attention and reap financial benefits, or in the course of deep psychological or psychiatric problems. In this section, we have presented several examples of these types of wounds, some of which are very dramatic. In our experience, clinicians are slow to recognize factitial wounds and, understandably, afraid to miss an important but unusual condition. When faced with a non-healing or unusual wound, there is a tendency to assume that either the proper treatments have not been used or that the diagnosis is elusive and perhaps too difficult. We suggest that in these situations of failure to heal and no clear diagnosis, the opposite approach be used; we must be thinking of factitial disease while doing everything possible to arrive at alternative diagnoses. When using this approach, one can make use of wound-associated clues to factitial ulcers, in addition to paying attention to the patient's personality and associated medical problems. Ulcers characterized by a linear or geometric configuration and unusual location, and with a discrepancy between severe pain and rather insignificant clinical appearance, are suspect. As shown in this section, we make use of the Unna boot or other compression bandages to cover ulcers on the extremities which might be factitial and which do not seem to be venous in etiology. Improvement, while not necessarily proving that the ulcer is factitial, is helpful in management and suggestive of the possibility of some extrinsic factors.

While we have learned a considerable amount about the acute stages of classical wound repair (e.g. after scalpel surgery or burns), we know relatively little about the course of events following non-scalpel cosmetic approaches such as dermabrasion, laser treatment, and chemical peels. The available information is at the histologic level for the most part, with a paucity of knowledge about the cellular and molecular events which might be associated with these particular physical modalities. However, there is considerable interest in this area of research, and the next several years will surely witness more progress in this field. From the clinical standpoint, we need to understand better what causes and controls pigmentary changes after cutaneous injury. Control of scarring is just as important, and it would be beneficial to know more about how occlusion seems to downregulate the fibrotic response.

Clinical points

- Pretreatment with topical retinoic acid for a few weeks can speed up the rate of healing of wounds created by dermabrasion.
- Occlusion of wounds made with lasers or with dermabrasion accelerates resurfacing and may decrease scarring.
- Low-potency topical steroids can help reduce the inflammation following TCA peels.
- Pretreatment with bleaching creams may decrease the chance of hyperpigmentation following a TCA peel.
- Occlusive dressings decrease postoperative pain and make the patient more comfortable.

- Adherent foam dressings are emerging as the dressings of choice after laser resurfacing procedures.
- The concomitant or recent use of oral isotretinoin is associated with the occurrence of exuberant granulation tissue after skin surgery.
- Trauma or surgical procedures in areas of skin which have previously (even years earlier) received gamma irradiation are often associated with non-healing wounds.
- Persistent redness or dermatitis after laser resurfacing may respond to topical or systemic steroids.
- A net-like (livedo) pattern surrounding a wound may have been caused by heat injury.
- A topical triple anesthetic (EMLA) can help relieve pain in certain wounds caused by trauma, such as burn or chemical injury.
- Factitial ulcers can often be managed by shielding the affected area with dressings or compression bandages.
- Warfarin (coumadin) necrosis is associated with protein C deficiency.
- Gamma irradiation is probably associated with persistent abnormalities in the phenotype of skin cells in the field of injury.
- Extensive fluoroscopy is associated with skin changes resembling radiation injury.

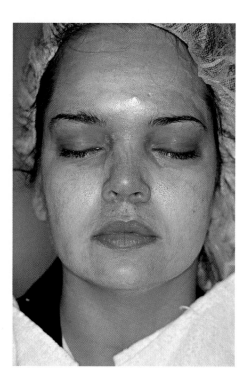

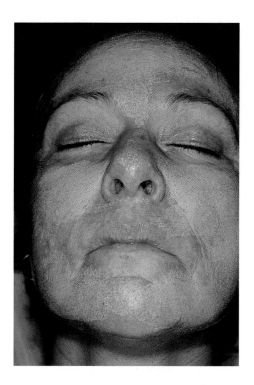

Figure 1.1
Trichloroacetic acid (TCA) peel

A 35% trichloroacetic acid peel is considered a mid-depth peel. The frosting seen here will last less than 15 min. This type of injury is characterized by redness, followed by peeling of the epidermis and upper dermis over a 1-week period. Skin care after a TCA peel consists of the use of moisturizers and, occasionally, a low-potency topical steroid to reduce inflammation. Pretreatment with topical retinoic acid and bleaching creams may speed up the healing and reduce the occurrence of hyperpigmentation, respectively.

Figure 1.2a
Trichloroacetic acid (TCA) peel

Again, here one sees the frosting immediately after the application of 35% TCA. Patients will often complain of stinging which, if severe, can be blocked by neutralizing the TCA with cold water. Sometimes, it is difficult to apply the same amount evenly, as this case illustrates. One often tries to avoid apposing surfaces around the nose.

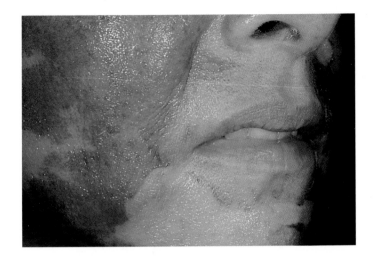

Figure 1.2b
Trichloroacetic acid (TCA) peel/Follow-up

This photograph was taken 4 days later. At this time, one can see that some of the skin is still dark due to the acid injury, while in other areas, such as the chin, peeling has already occurred. Because of this variation in skin pigmentation during the early stages (usually a week) of TCA peels, patients should be warned that their skin may look unsightly for a while.

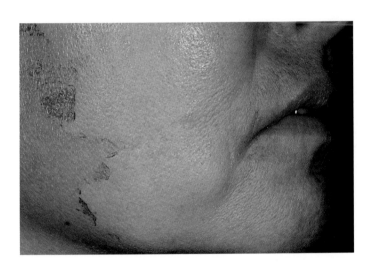

Figure 1.2c
Trichloroacetic acid (TCA) peel/Follow-up

This is 7 days after the peel. One can see that most of the treated skin has peeled off, and that the skin now looks healthier with a more pink complexion.

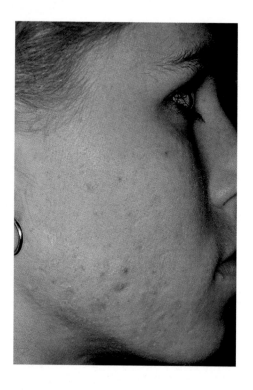

Figure 1.3a
Dermabrasion

A patient with acne scars can be improved either with dermabrasion or laser resurfacing. If the patient, like this one, has fair skin and light eyes, then resurfacing just the scar areas may be performed with less fear of ending up with areas of pigment demarcation. Pretreatment for 4 weeks with topical retinoic acid has been shown to increase the rate of re-epithelialization after resurfacing.

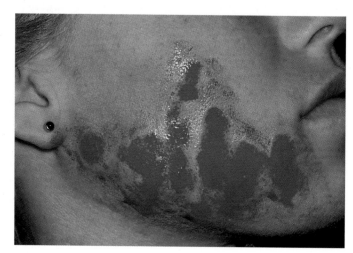

Figure 1.3b
Dermabrasion/After procedure

The picture was taken immediately after dermabrasion of the acne scars. Dermabrasion creates a partial-thickness wound. The dermabrasion was accomplished with a power dermabrader after the application of a skin refrigerant. In such cases, hemostasis is achieved with about 10 min of constant pressure. Following the procedure, the wound was treated with a topical antibiotic ointment and a hydrogel occlusive dressing, an occlusive regimen which speeds up healing and makes the patient more comfortable.

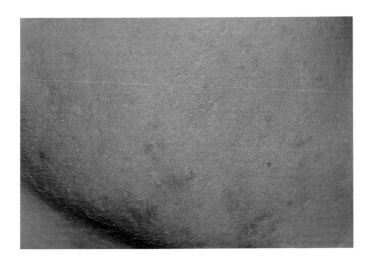

Figure 1.3c
Dermabrasion/Follow-up

The photograph was taken some months later. No persistent erythema or pigment demarcation lines are noted postoperatively. In general, dermabrasion creates less postoperative erythema than laser resurfacing because of less thermal damage.

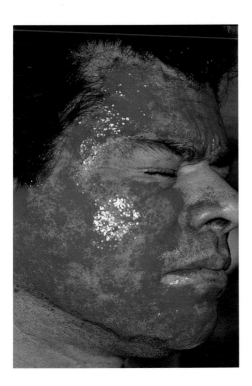

Figure 1.4
Full-face dermabrasion

Treatment of this extensive partial-thickness wound can be greatly facilitated by the use of an occlusive environment. This can be accomplished with the frequent application of ointments or with occlusive dressings. The non-dermabraded areas can be treated with 35% trichloroacetic acid (TCA) so that there is nice blending without a pigment demarcation line. Pain can be substantial after dermabrasion and may require narcotics for management. The pain is caused by the skin being wounded and exposed. Thus, occlusive dressing therapy, such as hydrogels, are helpful.

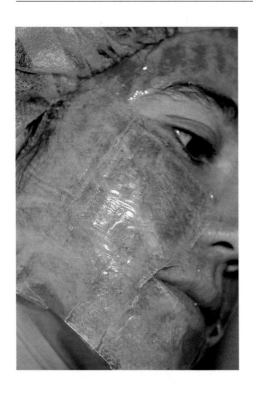

Figure 1.5
Dermabrasion

Here one can see a hydrogel covering the dermabraded areas. The hydrogel dressing can greatly reduce pain and speed up the rate of healing. Usually, the hydrogel dressing is kept in place over the wound with a stockinette netting similar to those used on extremities. The dressing usually needs to be changed every 24 h because of the abundant exudate, which tends to dislodge it. Patients can also obtain comfort and instant relief if the hydrogel is slightly cooled prior to application to the dermabraded wound.

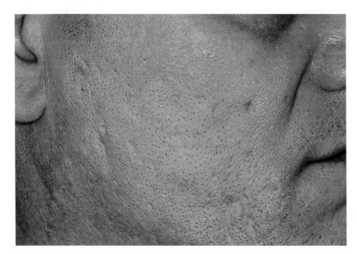

Figure 1.6
Dermabrasion/Hypopigmentation

The use of skin refrigerant has been implicated as a cause of hypopigmentation after dermabrasion. One hypothesis is that the skin refrigerant causes injury to the melanocytes. Hypopigmentation is also seen after laser resurfacing where the dwell time of pulse duration is greater than 900 µs; this pulse duration may lead to greater thermal damage than what is observed with shorter pulsed carbon dioxide lasers. There is no optimal way to improve the hypopigmentation, but camouflaged cosmetics are commonly used for that purpose.

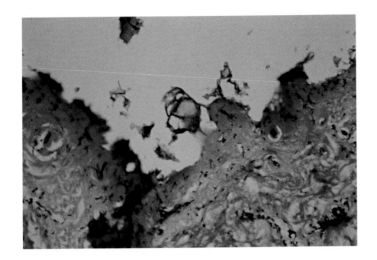

Figure 1.7
Thermal damage from laser

This photomicrograph shows evidence of thermal injury to the dermis following treatment with a carbon dioxide laser used with a computer scanning device that creates a dwell time of 950 µs. This duration, representing less than the thermal relaxation time of tissue, should create less heat diffusion to surrounding tissue than the previous generation of continuous carbon dioxide lasers. This photomicrograph demonstrates coagulation necrosis of the epidermis and dermis. Thrombosis of blood vessels, dilatation of adjacent blood vessels and interstitial fluid leading to edema, weeping and oozing may also be seen.

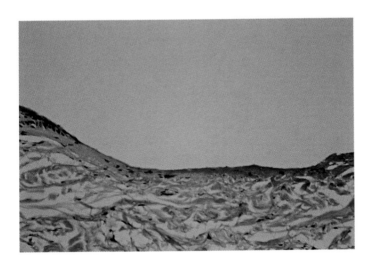

Figure 1.8
Thermal damage from laser

Generally, much less thermal damage is created by a shorter pulse duration laser (90µs pulse duration), although in the case shown here the laser was used to create ablation at about the same depth as the previous photomicrograph. The shorter pulse duration lasers also cause less postoperative erythema.

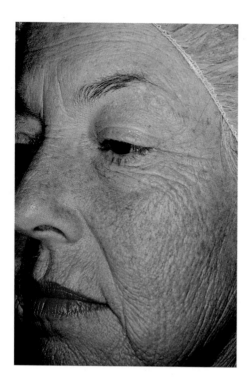

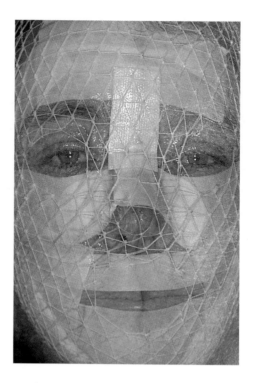

Figure 1.9a
Laser resurfacing

This patient has severe wrinkling from sun damage. To improve the appearance of her skin, one could use any of the carbon dioxide lasers. Realistically, the best results can probably be expected around her mouth and eyes. As in most cases, the patient was pretreated with topical retinoic acid and bleaching creams. The retinoic acid appears to speed up the rate of healing. Bleaching creams (i.e. 4% hydroquinone) tend to decrease the occurrence of postoperative hyperpigmentation. As a general rule, patients undergoing this procedure are also started on an antiviral medication such as acyclovir, valacyclovir, or famciclovir, to minimize the occurrence of postoperative herpes simplex infection.

Figure 1.9b
Laser resurfacing (postoperative dressing)

The advantages of using a foam type of occlusive dressing for the first 3 days after laser resurfacing are greater absorption of blood and exudate, less pain, faster healing, and easier wound care for the patient.

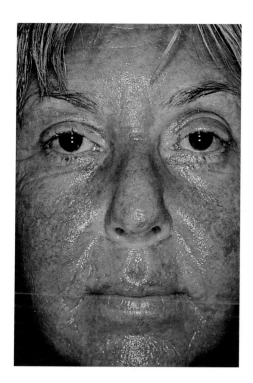

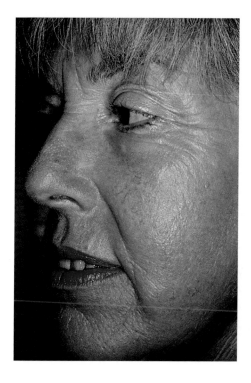

Figure 1.9c
Laser resurfacing (follow-up)

This photograph was taken 4 days later. The resurfacing was done with the laser used at 500 mJ 90 μsec pulse duration and with six passes over most areas of the face except the eyes, where only three passes were used. The picture was taken immediately after the removal of the foam (adherent) occlusive dressing.

Figure 1.9d
Laser resurfacing (follow-up)

This photograph was taken 1 month after the procedure. The results are quite good. There appears to be substantial improvement of the wrinkles around her mouth. It is thought that shrinkage of the dermis and collagenous component by the laser treatment accounts for much of the early cosmetic improvement. There was less thermal damage and less postoperative erythema in this patient compared with other patients who have had laser resurfacing.

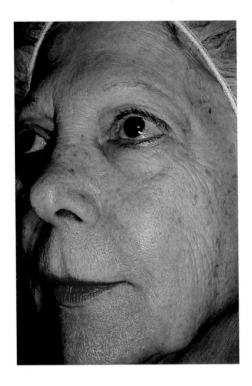

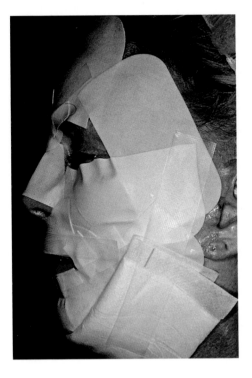

Figure 1.10a
Laser resurfacing

Preoperative photograph of a patient about
to undergo laser resurfacing of her face.
Unlike the previous case, there appears to be
less sun damage to her skin and the majority
of her wrinkles are away from her mouth.

Figure 1.10b
Laser resurfacing (postoperative dressing)

Again, adherent foam occlusive dressings, as
used in this case as well, appear to be the
dressing of choice in many laser resurfacing
procedures. The dressing is applied over the
entire wounded area by overlapping. Any
wound covered with an occlusive dressing
goes through an early exudative phase.
Therefore, it is wise to use an absorbent
dressing around the chin, where the exudate
will collect due to gravity. A netting
stockinette is placed over the dressing to
keep it in place over the wound.

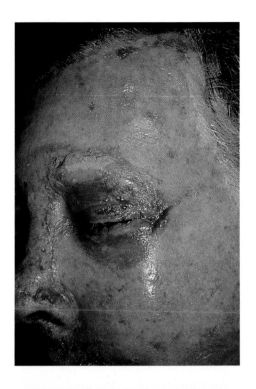

Figure 1.10c
Laser resurfacing/5 days later

The resurfacing was done with a 90-μs pulse duration carbon dioxide laser. There is more exudate, crusting, and erythema around the non-occluded areas compared with the areas where the wound was treated with the occlusive dressing.

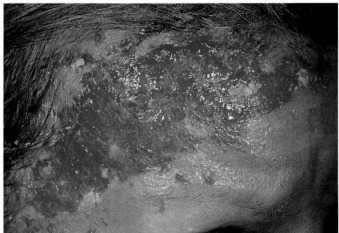

Figure 1.11
History of prior radiation exposure

Here, unfortunately, laser resurfacing was done in an area that had received gamma radiation more than 30 years earlier for the treatment of acne. The damage from radiation is longstanding, and wounds created over these areas do not heal readily. In addition to prior radiation exposure, another but more relative contraindication to laser resurfacing is the recent use of isotretinoin. The latter has been associated with the formation of exuberant granulation tissue. The laser procedure in this case was done with normal parameters using a 950-μs pulse duration carbon dioxide laser and a computer scanner. Six months after the procedure, her skin was still not healed.

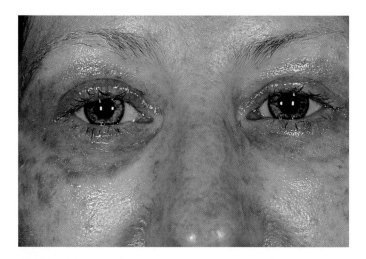

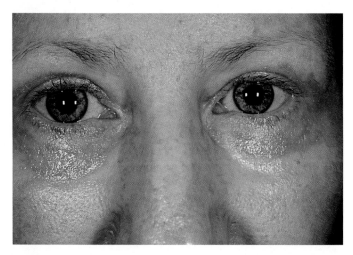

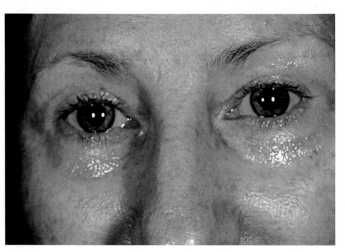

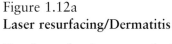

Figure 1.12a
Laser resurfacing/Dermatitis

Ten days after laser resurfacing, an apparent irritant or allergic contact dermatitis developed in non-wounded and non-occluded areas treated with a topical antibiotic (bacitracin ointment).

Figure 1.12b
Laser resurfacing/Dermatitis

Weeks later, the patient still had redness around her eyes. No further antibiotic ointments had been applied, and diagnostic considerations included a bacterial or candida infection, which could have been exacerbated by the use of the ointment and occlusion. This points to the difficulty of determining with certainty what happens during the postoperative period, when antibiotics and dressings are commonly used.

Figure 1.12c
Laser resurfacing/Dermatitis

This photograph was taken 6 months after the laser resurfacing procedure. As shown, the patient continues to have a persistent dermatitis. The problem finally resolved with the use of topical and systemic corticosteroids. The exact cause of the dermatitis was never determined.

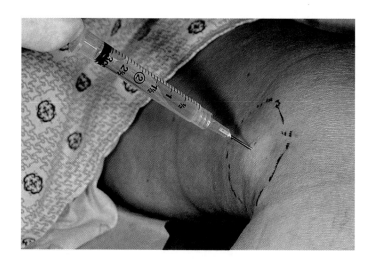

Figure 1.13
Seroma/Hematoma after liposuction

This patient developed a seroma after liposuction of the knee. The usual management of this complication involves drainage of the clear or serosanguinous fluid. Repeated drainage is often required.

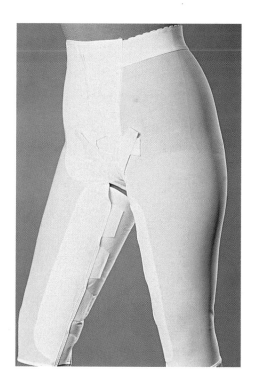

Figure 1.14
Compression garment

Compression garments may decrease the incidence of hematomas or seromas. These garments are worn by patients for at least 1 week after liposuction.

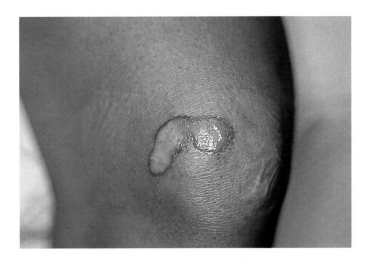

Figure 1.15a
Traumatic wound

This was caused by a fall and became quite painful. The surface of the wound is yellow-white, suggesting bacterial contamination. However, there is no evidence of cellulitis.

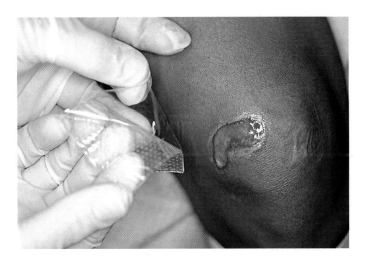

Figure 1.15b
Traumatic wound/Pain management

Gel dressings are ideal for this type of superficial but painful wound. These types of dressings are usually made of a polyethylene gel-like material sandwiched between two polyurethane films. Only the polyurethane film from the dressing side in contact with the wound is removed.

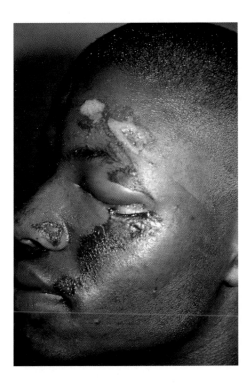

Figure 1.16
Traumatic wound

This photograph was taken 2 days after the patient reported falling onto gravel. There is a great deal of swelling, bruising and superficial skin loss on the forehead, cheeks, and nose. Generally, this type of injury heals without scarring, although keloid formation and tattooing are definite possibilities.

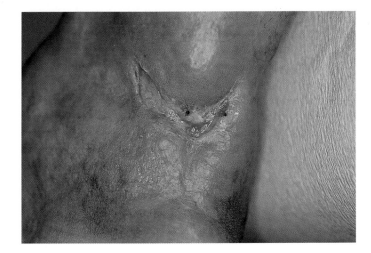

Figure 1.17
Non-healing traumatic wound

This patient had a surgical procedure to repair her Achilles tendon. Postoperatively, she was placed in a cast to immobilize her leg. This type of laceration just above the heel was present after the cast was removed and has not healed for several months. There is considerable induration and probable fibrosis around this wound. As in other situations like this, the fibrotic component may be interfering with the healing process. Topical retinoic acid, used to stimulate granulation tissue, did not improve this wound. She was lost to follow-up, but our plan was to excise the fibrotic tissue around the wound, followed by grafting.

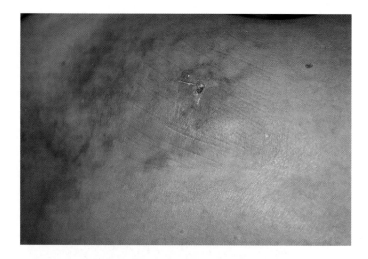

Figure 1.18a
Burn injury

This area on the left flank and back shows a livedo pattern (erythema ab igne) and ulceration. The patient had been applying a heating pad to this site in order to relieve back pain. This is a not uncommon clinical situation, particularly in the elderly. The livedo presumably represents damage to the superficial vasculature.

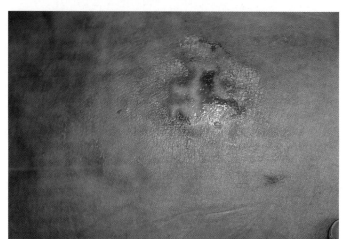

Figure 1.18b
Burn injury/Close-up

The ulceration is surrounded by the livedo pattern and appears to be quite superficial. It healed with the use of occlusive dressings.

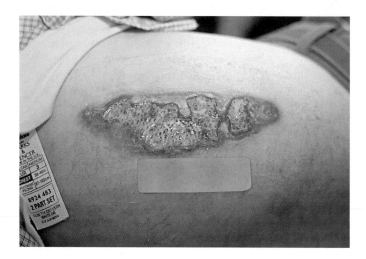

Figure 1.19
Electrocautery burn

A partial thickness skin loss with a combination of active granulation tissue epithelialization and slough occurring together.

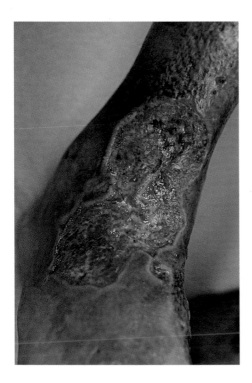

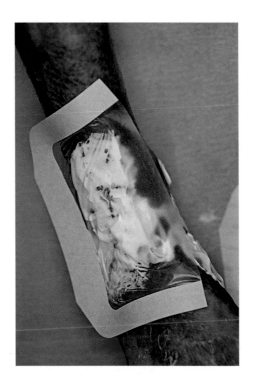

Figure 1.20a
Wound from chemical injury

This patient was injured by exposure to a chemical while at work. These and other wounds on his feet did not heal in spite of a number of therapeutic approaches. Pain is a persistent problem. The patient also had cirrhosis. Although the chemical injury may have been the inciting event, his clinical picture was one of venous insufficiency. Generally, he tended to improve with compression therapy.

Figure 1.20b
Wound from chemical injury/Pain control

Persistent pain was this patient's greatest problem. In this and in other chronic wounds, we have found that a topical triple anesthetic that is commercially available (EMLA cream) is quite effective in relieving pain. Here one sees the cream that has been placed on the wound and is being covered with a semi-occlusive film (the paper support for the film is yet to be removed). The use of the film is probably not necessary, because there is good absorption of the EMLA cream in wounds.

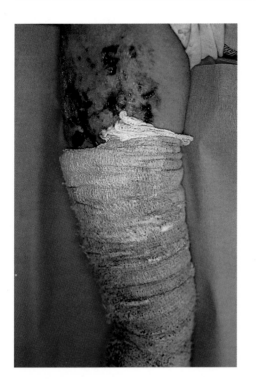

Figure 1.21a
Factitial ulcers

This patient had a number of recurrent necrotic ulcerations on the right forearm. Histologic and laboratory studies did not show any evidence of vasculitis, cryoglobulinemia, cryofibrinogenemia, or antiphospholipid syndrome. The patient admitted that she was extensively scratching and picking her skin. In our experience this type of problem is linked to psychiatric disease. It was decided to shield the area from further trauma by applying an Unna boot to the arm, from the wrist to the elbow. However, as shown in the photograph, the bandage had a tendency to slip down, possibly as a result of further manipulation by the patient.

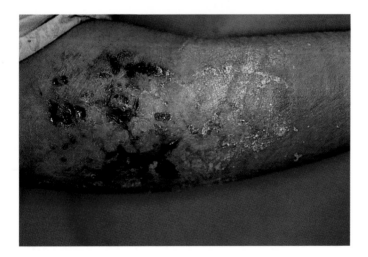

Figure 1.21b
Factitial ulcers/Close-up

Here the Unna boot has just been removed and it can be seen that the inferior area still protected by the bandage has healed. This told us that we were on the right track, both diagnostically and therapeutically.

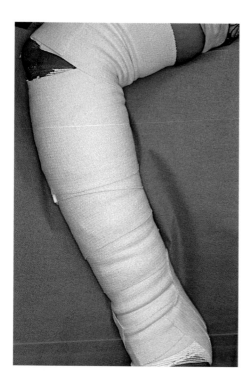

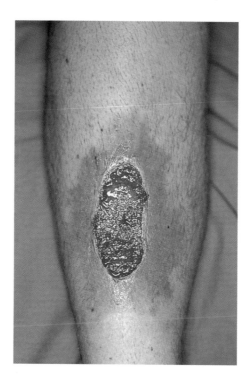

Figure 1.21c
Factitial ulcers/Treatment with bandage

We realized that a modification of the bandaging was needed to anchor the Unna boot in place. This was successfully achieved by applying the Unna boot from the upper arm to the wrist and then cutting a section over the elbow. This allowed the patient more freedom of movement and helped to ensure greater compliance. The patient healed and, interestingly, did not continue to injure her arm.

Figure 1.22a
Factitial leg ulcers

This 32-year-old woman cannot stop producing these large ulcers. She clearly admits to it but says that she cannot stop when she gets the urge to damage her skin. It is unclear how she produces these ulcers. She denies using sharp objects and says that she simply keeps rubbing her skin off. Dressings have been of no value, and protecting the skin with bandages (like an Unna boot) has not worked. She easily removes all bandages.

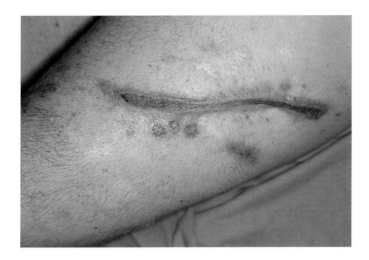

Figure 1.22b
Factitial leg ulcers/Linear lesion on the thigh

This is the same patient with a large linear ulceration on her thigh and some smaller ulcers around it. This large ulcer seems to have been produced with a sharp object. The plan is to treat the patient with pimozide, which is usually reserved for patients with delusional parasitosis but has worked in some patients with factitial ulcers. Sleep studies were normal and did not show EEG abnormalities or bouts of destructive behavior while the patient was asleep.

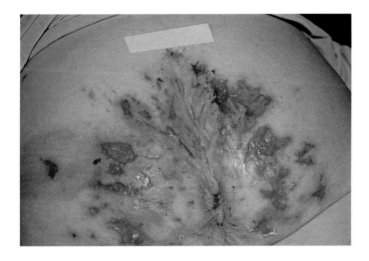

Figure 1.23
Factitial perianal ulcers

These extensive ulcers and erosions were caused by the patient, who suffered from dementia. There was no evidence of infection with herpes simplex viruses. The possibility of zinc deficiency was entertained, but there was no other periorificial involvement or evidence for zinc deficiency. Extensive use of hydrocolloids is probably the best way to protect these areas from further manipulation.

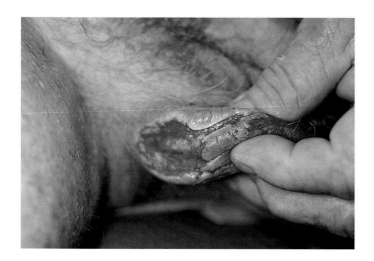

Figure 1.24
Factitial scrotal ulcer

Often, there is very little one can do for factitial ulcers. He has recurrent scrotal ulcers that, clinically, appear to be due to external injury. He denied self harm, but after evaluation (biopsies, cultures) our clinical judgment is that these are self-inflicted wounds. Patients like this generally refuse to be evaluated by a psychiatrist.

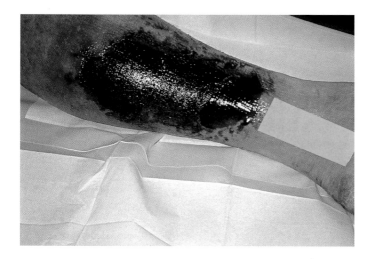

Figure 1.25
Warfarin (coumadin) necrosis

This is a well-known complication in patients on warfarin. It is thought to be due to protein C deficiency during the initial phases of therapy with warfarin.

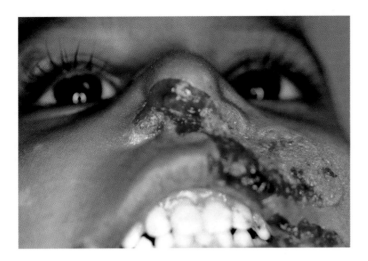

Figure 1.26a
Junctional epidermolysis bullosa

This condition became apparent a week after birth and has plagued this child ever since. The variant shown here (Herlitz variant) is characterized by excessive granulation tissue and lesions often occurring on the face. Scarring is the norm. In this case, the excessive granulation tissue has led to obliteration of the nares. These patients may also suffer from gastrointestinal involvement. All forms of junctional epidermolysis bullosa are characterized by cleavage through the lamina lucida.

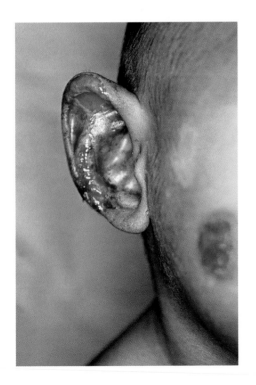

Figure 1.26b
Junctional epidermolysis bullosa

He also had wounds on his ears. A serious management problem in these patients is bleeding, which occurs readily as soon as the wound is touched or dressed. Trauma is important in the development of these wounds. We found petrolatum-impregnated gauze to be the best dressing for most of his wounds.

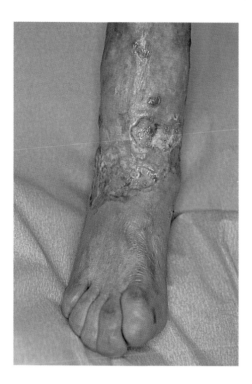

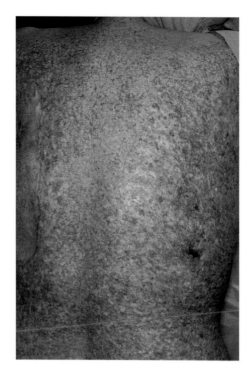

Figure 1.27
Dystrophic epidermolysis bullosa

This picture was taken when the patient was 63 years old. He first developed the condition at the age of 2. The pattern of inheritance was autosomal dominant. The cleavage and blister formation in this disease is below the lamina densa. Basically, the clinical course here is one of chronic wounds. However, trauma plays a major role in the development of these wounds.

Figure 1.28a
Radiation-induced wounds

This patient had cutaneous T-cell lymphoma and received total body electron beam therapy several years earlier. The lymphoma appears to be under control. However, the radiation has caused the skin to become atrophic. Areas of skin breakdown became a management problem.

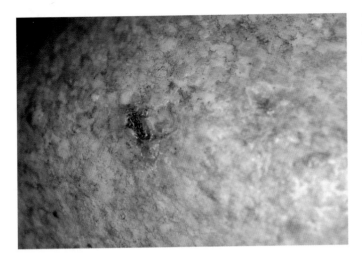

Figure 1.28b
Radiation-induced wounds/Close-up

This patient's skin is indurated, and shows remarkable apparent vascularity, which is probably due to blood vessel damage and tortuosity as well as vascular proliferation. These superficial wounds were very painful, and did not respond to a variety of occlusive dressings or to topical retinoic acid. Topical steroids appear to improve the symptoms in some of these patients. In our opinion, the epidermal and dermal cells are damaged by the radiation and are altered in a fundamental way. One hope is to use autologous grafting or bioengineered skin to re-establish a normal cell population.

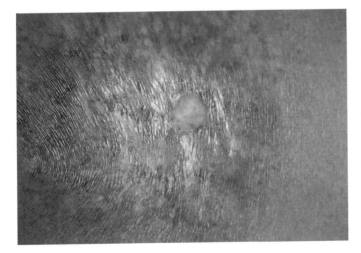

Figure 1.29
Fluoroscopy-induced wound

This complication of intense exposure to X-rays during prolonged fluoroscopic procedures is not well recognized among radiologists or other clinicians. In this case, the patient had had a liver transplant and many fluoroscopic procedures. This indurated lesion on his back with a central non-healing ulcer was initially thought to be morphea by his physicians. However, the vascular and pigmented lesion is most compatible with radiation-induced damage. He was helped by medium-potency topical steroid, which markedly reduced his pain. A full-thickness graft taken from his thigh took initially but did not survive long term. We suspect that the intense immunosuppression from corticosteroids and cyclosporin also played a large role in preventing healing.

2 Acute wounds: surgical

Introduction

In the previous section, we have discussed rather superficial wounds caused by trauma or sugical injury by lasers, chemicals, and dermabrasion. As mentioned, we often make the assumption that those types of wounds follow a pattern of repair that is similar to that of acute wounds created by scalpel. That may not be the case. In this section, we discuss acute wounds, such as those caused by the surgeon to remove skin cancer, to repair a surgical defect or scar, or to treat some chronic conditions, such as hidradenitis suppurativa. It is likely that in these types of surgical wounds the cellular and molecular events we have learned about in the last few years are more applicable. Therefore, before we outline this section, it would be helpful to briefly review the fundamentals of wound repair after acute injury.

For the purpose of facilitating understanding and for communication of concepts, the wound repair process is generally divided into the three phases of inflammation, fibroplasia, and maturation. Overlap between these phases is considerable, however. The inflammatory phase occurs immediately after the types of acute injury described in this section. Platelets enter the wound and release a host of mediators which recruit other cell types and amplify the initial response. In addition to a number of biochemical signals (e.g. fibrinogen, thrombospondin, and thromboxane A_2, ADP), a variety of growth factors are released, including platelet-derived growth factor (PDGF), transforming growth factor-β_1 (TGF-β_1), and connective tissue growth factor (CTGF). The formation of a thrombus leads to the release of other inflammatory molecules, such as bradykinin, C3a and C3b, which enhance vascular permeability. Ultimately, this phase of wound repair is characterized by platelet release and clot formation, wound debridement by neutrophils, and recruitment of macrophages, fibroblasts, and endothelial cells.

Macrophages, fibroblasts, and endothelial cells play a fundamental role in the second (proliferative) phase of wound repair. Collagen and other structural molecules are laid down, and the dermal matrix is reconstituted. Granulation tissue is formed. Angiogenesis takes place while the matrix make-up of the wound keeps changing. In turn, the change in matrix alters the angiogenic response. Certain growth factors, such as vascular endothelial growth factor (VEGF) and fibroblast growth factors (FGFs), are key components of the angiogenic response. Integrins, cell surface receptor molecules, are important in facilitating the interactions between cells and matrix and in cell migration, including that of keratinocytes.

Tissue remodelling represents the third and final phase of wound repair. This phase may go on for weeks, perhaps months, and is characterized by the presence and activity of a host of enzymes able to break down matrix components. The matrix-degrading metalloproteinases (MMPs) comprise three broad classes (collagenases, gelatinases, and stromelysins). These enzymes, which need to be activated to function, have a certain amount of specificity for different collagens and other matrix proteins. At the same time, fibroblasts continue to synthesize extracellular matrix components. Therefore, tissue formation and remodelling go on at the same time.

The above is obviously a very brief summary and overview of what follows injury to the skin. However, it outlines the processes which occur following most of the surgical procedures described in this section. To the extent that one can modify the wound repair response, one might obtain different and perhaps more desirable clinical results. We do not know how to control fibrosis yet, although experimental approaches to block the action of certain growth factors (e.g. TGF-βs) seem promising. At least in more superficial wounds, occlusive dressings may downregulate the fibrotic response. They also create the moist wound environment which accelerates healing of acute wounds. Full-thickness grafts can be used to minimize contraction. As also discussed in the previous section, topical pretreatment of skin with retinoic acid might be able to accelerate healing of acute wounds, but this approach has not been properly tested for standard scalpel-induced wounds. This section shows a number of examples where the location of the wound on the face dictates the extent of contraction. For example, wounds in concave areas of the face (versus convex) seem to heal better by secondary intention. The cellular and molecular events underlying these observations are unknown. However, knowing these clinical parameters is important, because it alters our surgical approach.

It should be noted that a number of examples given in this section are related to Mohs surgery for removal of skin cancer. However, the lessons learned are not restricted to this specific surgical procedure. We should simply think of these as wounds as being created by the scalpel and, in some cases, left to heal by secondary intention. The use of dressings, postoperative care, scarring and contraction are important clinical components that are applicable to other types of wounds as well. Indeed, facial wounds, such as those created by Mohs micrographic surgery, provide a special window into how the repair process occurs in humans, and have led to observations regarding the healing of convex versus concave areas of the face.

Clinical points

• Tensile strength after complete wound repair can only be as high as 70% of that of uninjured skin.
• In secondary intention healing, concave areas of the face heal with less scarring than those in convex areas.
• Scalp ulcerations, for example after skin cancer surgery, are often difficult to heal if there has been a lot of actinic damage.
• Mohs surgery is quite effective in removing skin cancer completely, while sparing as much non-cancerous tissue as possible.
• Bioengineered skin can be used to speed up healing of facial Mohs surgery defects.
• The optimal time for dermabrasion or laser resurfacing for postoperative scars is about 2 months after surgery.
• The treatment of extensive and long-standing hidradenitis suppurativa generally involves extensive surgery to remove the apocrine glands and draining sinuses.
• Beefy red granulation tissue is not necessarily healthy and may signify bacterial overgrowth.
• Occlusive dressings are an established way to accelerate healing of acute wounds. The fear of infection associated with occlusive dressings is unwarranted.

- Redness of healed wounds can last for up to a year.

- Calcium alginate dressings can be useful in absorbing exudate.

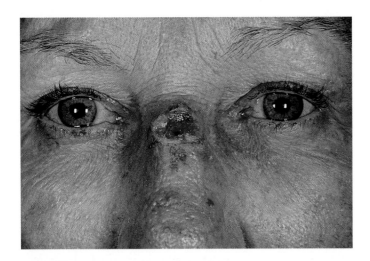

Figure 2.1a
Ulcer from cryosurgery

A wound caused by cryosurgery usually starts as a hemorrhagic blister, followed by ulceration and crusting. The surrounding tissue can become quite edematous. In this patient, liquid nitrogen had been used to treat an actinic keratosis.

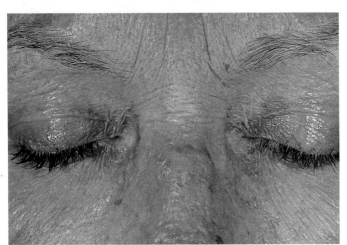

Figure 2.1b
Ulcer from cryosurgery/Follow-up

The wound has healed completely. In other cases, healing is complicated by substantial hypopigmentation, presumably because of damage to melanocytes.

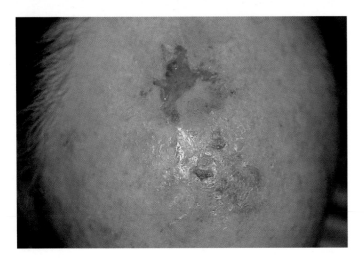

Figure 2.2a
Non-healing scalp ulcerations

After removal of a widespread basal cell carcinoma, the resulting surgical wound was left to heal by secondary intention. However, complete healing did not occur over a period of several months. This is not an uncommon problem after surgery in actinically damaged, fragile skin.

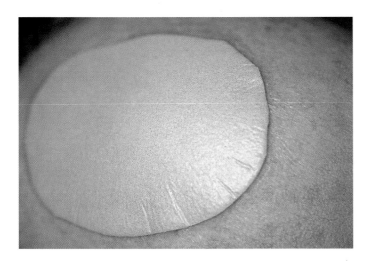

Figure 2.2b
Non-healing scalp ulcerations/Treatment with a hydrocolloid

This therapy is beneficial because the moist wound healing environment created by these dressings accelerates healing. Also, the dressing protects the wound from further injury. Manufacturers of these dressings recommend removing or changing them at least weekly. However, in selected cases where there is little drainage we have found that they can stay on much longer. Indeed, removal of these adherent dressings can by itself cause further disruption of the epithelium. In this patient the hydrocolloid dressing was kept on the scalp for at least 2 weeks.

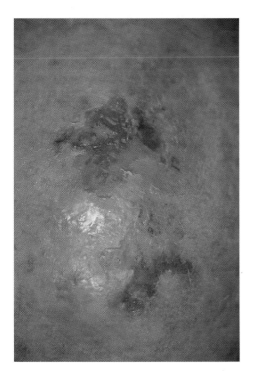

Figure 2.2c
Non-healing scalp ulcerations/After removal of the dressing

As seen here, there is now evidence of re-epithelialization and almost complete healing.

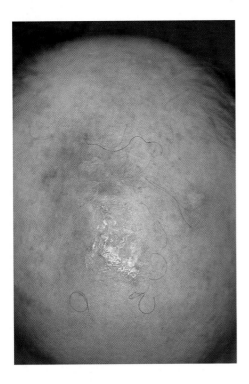

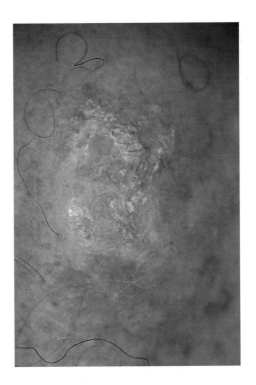

Figure 2.2d
Non-healing scalp ulcerations/Follow-up

There is now complete healing of the ulcerations, several months after starting treatment with the hydrocolloid dressing. This prolonged clinical course is not unusual in our experience.

Figure 2.2e
Non-healing scalp ulcerations/Close-up

This photograph shows that, although there is complete healing, the skin is still rather fragile and susceptible to injury from minor trauma.

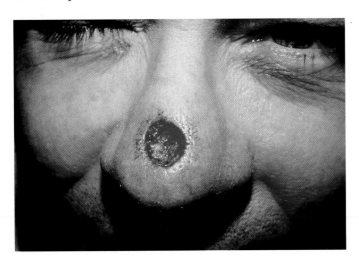

Figure 2.3a
Nasal wound after Mohs surgery

A full-thickness nasal wound, as shown here, should be repaired rather than left to heal by secondary intention. This is because convex areas of skin on the face heal rather poorly and with unsightly results by secondary intention.

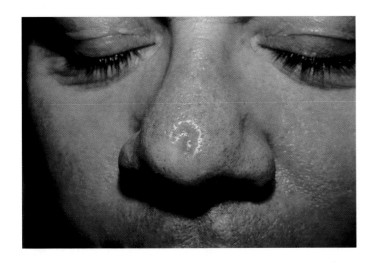

Figure 2.3b
Nasal wound after Mohs surgery/Scar

The resultant depressed scar will need to be repaired. Full-thickness skin grafts are often used for this purpose.

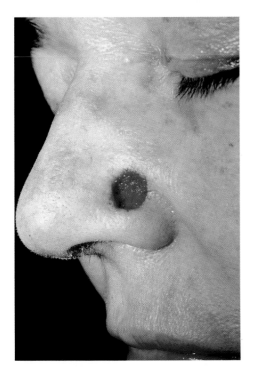

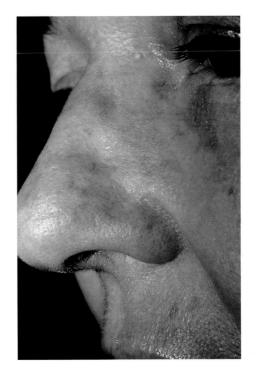

Figure 2.4a
Nasal defect after Mohs surgery

Unlike the situation in the previous case, this wound in a concave area of skin can be expected to heal with acceptable scarring by secondary intention.

Figure 2.4b
Nasal defect after Mohs surgery/Follow-up

Excellent cosmetic result with secondary intention healing. (Photo courtesy of John Zitelli, MD.)

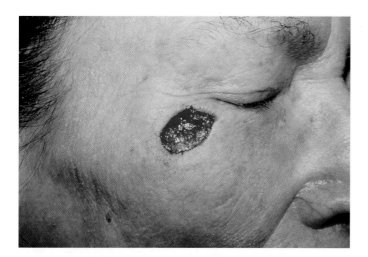

Figure 2.5a
Wound in a convex area

The wound is the result of removal of a skin cancer with Mohs surgery.

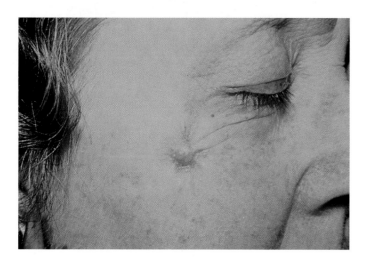

Figure 2.5b
Wound in convex area/Follow-up

As one might expect, secondary intention healing is not the appropriate way to treat these wounds over convex skin areas. There is considerable scarring and contraction.

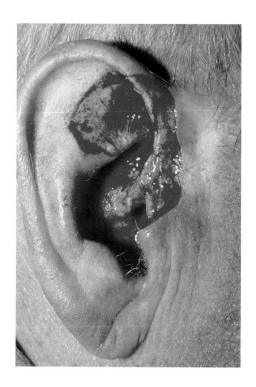

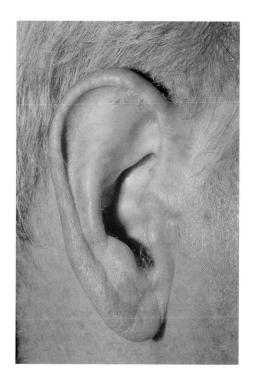

Figure 2.6a
Mohs surgery wound

Although it looks extensive, this type of ear wound heals quite well by secondary intention.

Figure 2.6b
Mohs surgery wound/Follow-up

Secondary intention healing in this area yields good cosmetic results.

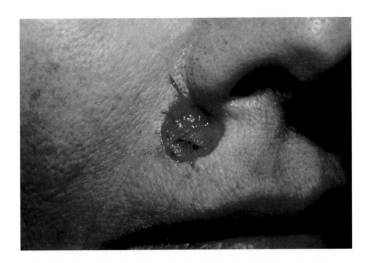

Figure 2.7a
Healing of Mohs wound

Skin cancers in these areas near the nasolabial folds can be very difficult to remove completely and have a high chance of recurrence. Mohs surgery, by microscopically ensuring complete removal of the cancer, is often the treatment of choice. This wound was allowed to heal by secondary intention.

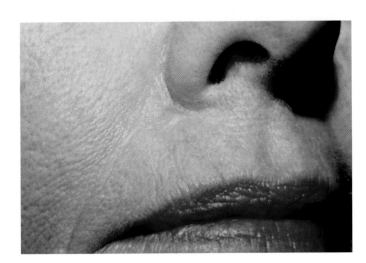

Figure 2.7b
Healing of Mohs wound/Follow-up

Small scar after healing by secondary intention. This result is acceptable to most patients because the scar is small. However, some clinicians would argue that a flap closure would have resulted in a better cosmetic outcome.

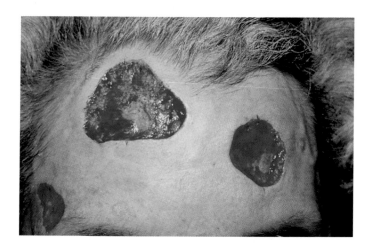

Figure 2.8a
Large and multiple Mohs wounds

Even these large wounds after Mohs surgery for skin cancer can heal well by secondary intention. Their management, particularly in the elderly, is very challenging. Although it has been shown that occlusive dressings will help these wounds heal faster, it has been our observation that most Mohs surgeons prefer to use topical antibiotics and non-adherent dressings and gauze in the initial phases. This preference may reflect concern over postoperative bleeding. One might argue that surgical repair of these wounds, rather than healing by secondary intention, should be done to minimize the patient's discomfort. A recent promising approach is the use of bioengineered skin.

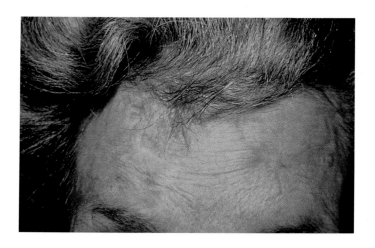

Figure 2.8b
Large and multiple Mohs wounds/Follow up

As shown here, the cosmetic results with secondary intention healing can be quite satisfactory. However, healing of these wounds required several months. The benefits and risks of repairing these large wounds surgically should be carefully evaluated.

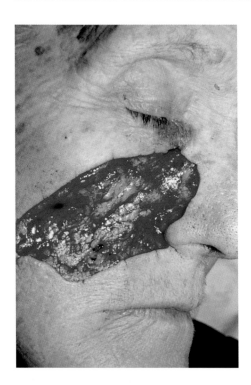

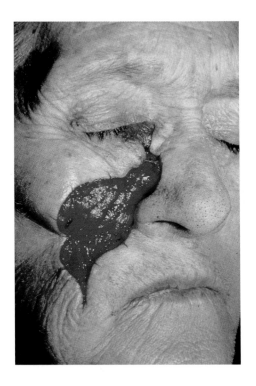

Figure 2.9a
Wound contraction

This wound on the cheek is the result of
Mohs surgery for skin cancer and could
cause an ectropion if allowed to heal by
secondary intention. The patient was given
several therapeutic options to minimize this
complication.

Figure 2.9b
Wound contraction/Follow-up

Horizontal (absorbable) guiding sutures were
used to partially pull the wound together, so
as to avoid a downward pull on the eyelid.

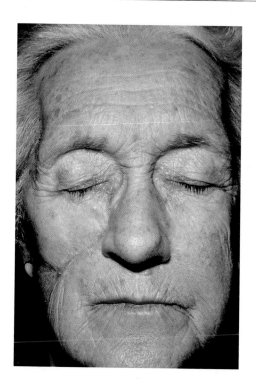

Figure 2.9c
Wound contraction/Follow-up

This photograph shows the final cosmetic result. There is no downward pull on the right lower eyelid and no functional impairment. This series of photographs show how a simple procedure can minimize the effects of wound contraction. Some patients, of course, would opt for more extensive surgical procedures that can yield better cosmetic results. (Courtesy of John Zitelli MD.)

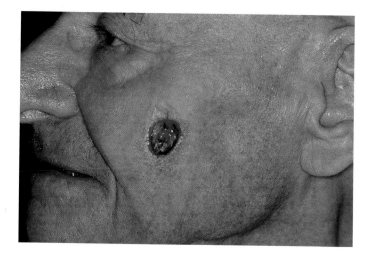

Figure 2.10a
Suturing of Mohs wound

This patient had a skin cancer treated by Mohs surgery. This full-thickness defect on the cheek should be sutured in order to achieve a good cosmetic result. Again, these convex areas do not heal well by secondary intention.

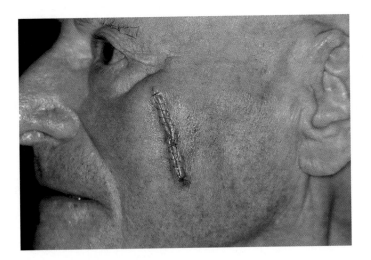

Figure 2.10b
Suturing of Mohs wound/Follow-up

If the wound is sutured flat, contraction will eventually create an indented scar. By suturing the wound with eversion of the edges, later contraction tends to lead to a flat scar and a more desirable cosmetic result.

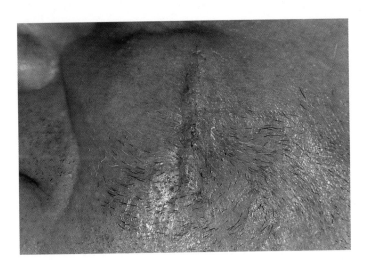

Figure 2.10c
Suturing of Mohs wound/Follow-up

Two months postoperatively showing an acceptable cosmetic result.

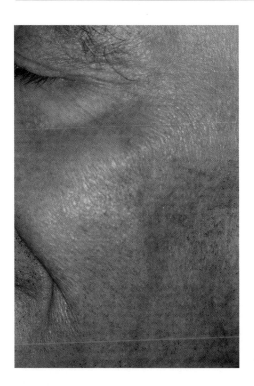

Figure 2.10d
Suturing of Mohs wound/Follow-up

Excellent cosmetic result several months later showing the extent of scar maturation over time.

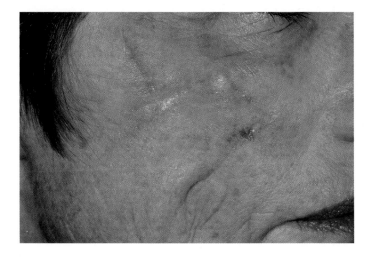

Figure 2.11a
Dog ear deformity

A rhombic flap on the cheek has created scars and dog ear deformity at the inferior margin. This picture was taken 2 weeks after surgical removal of a skin cancer.

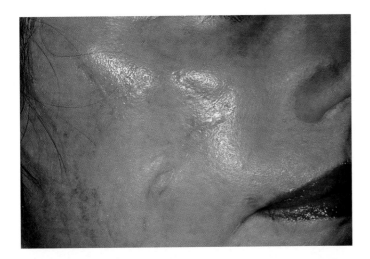

Figure 2.11b
Dog ear deformity/Follow-up

The appearance of the scar has improved 2 months postoperatively. The optimal time for dermabrasion or laser resurfacing to further improve the appearance of this type of scar is about 2 months after the flap procedure.

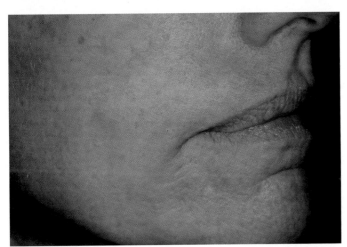

Figure 2.11c
Dog ear deformity/Follow-up

The scar was eventually resurfaced with a carbon dioxide laser. The appearance is quite acceptable.

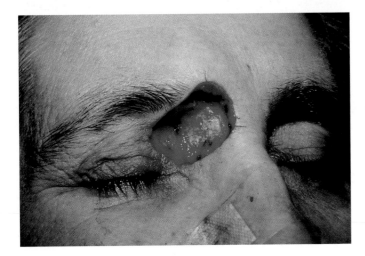

Figure 2.12a
Deep Mohs wound near the eyelid

Healing of this deep wound after removal of a skin cancer would most likely result in severe contraction and pulling of the upper eyelid upward. This complication would have both cosmetic and functional consequences.

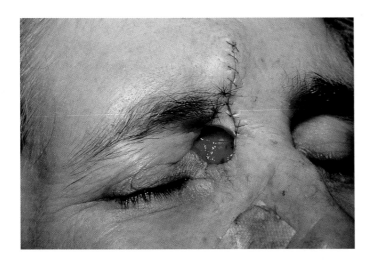

Figure 2.12b
Deep Mohs wound near the eyelid/Closure

The wound was closed primarily with the dog ear used as a full-thickness skin graft.

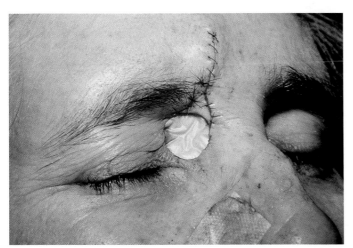

Figure 2.12c
Deep Mohs wound near the eyelid

A type I collagen matrix material was also used to fill the remaining defect. This type of matrix is thought to act as a scaffold for migrating fibroblasts and to decrease contraction.

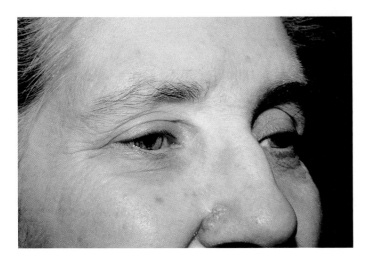

Figure 2.12d
Deep Mohs wound near the eyelid

The final result is quite pleasing. The lesion in the nasolabial fold is most likely another basal cell carcinoma which will require further surgery. (Courtesy of John Zitelli MD.)

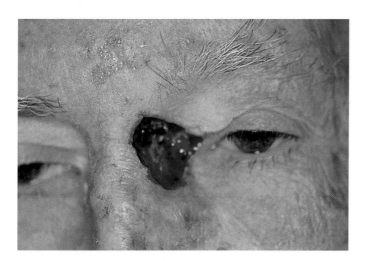

Figure 2.13a
Full-thickness Mohs wound

The wound is the result of Mohs surgery to remove a basal cell carcinoma in the medial canthal area. A full-thickness graft is a good way to repair this defect.

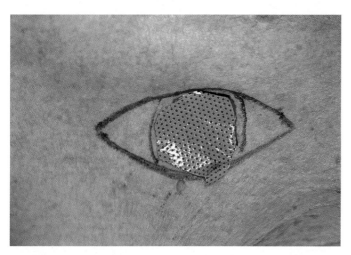

Figure 2.13b
Full-thickness Mohs wound/Donor site

The area directly over the clavicle is a good source of full-thickness grafts for larger facial wounds. A template is used to mark the donor site of the graft. A sterile dressing or other suitable material can be used as a template.

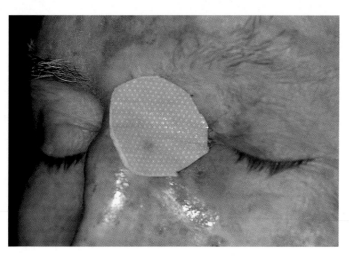

Figure 2.13c
Full-thickness Mohs wound/Grafted

A non-adherent bandage is placed over the full-thickness graft.

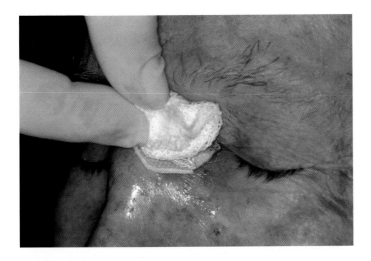

Figure 2.13d
Full-thickness Mohs wound/Grafted

Wadded-up gauze is used to maintain pressure over the graft and to minimize graft loss due to the accumulation of blood or wound fluid.

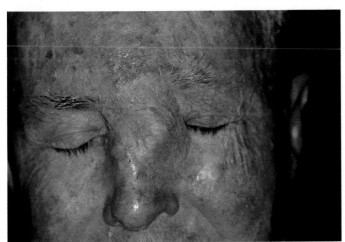

Figure 2.13e
Full-thickness Mohs wound/Grafted

Here one sees the pressure dressing in place, covered and secured with paper tape and liquid adhesive.

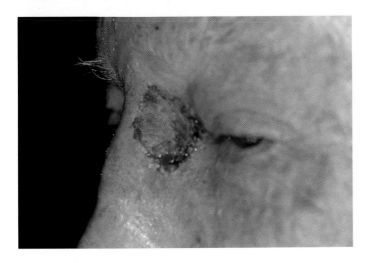

Figure 2.13f
Full-thickness Mohs wound/Follow-up

This photograph, taken 7 days after the procedure, shows excellent graft take.

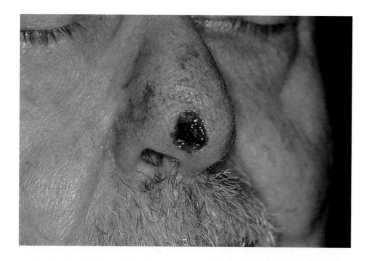

Figure 2.14a
Full-thickness wound/Nasal ala

This photograph was taken immediately after Mohs surgery to remove a basal cell carcinoma. This full-thickness wound near the nasal ala can cause alar rim distortion if left to heal by secondary intention.

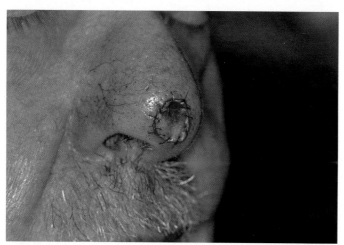

Figure 2.14b
Full-thickness wound/Nasal ala

A full-thickness graft was sutured into the wound. In this case, the donor site was the postauricular area.

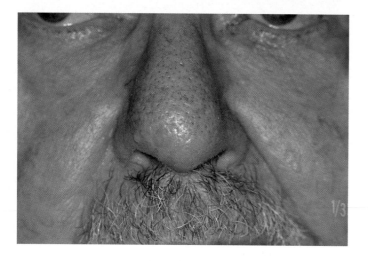

Figure 2.14c
Full-thickness wound/Nasal ala

As shown here, the final result was quite acceptable. The full-thickness graft was able to prevent wound contraction. It is important, when choosing the donor site, to match as closely as possible the skin color and texture of the skin around the defect.

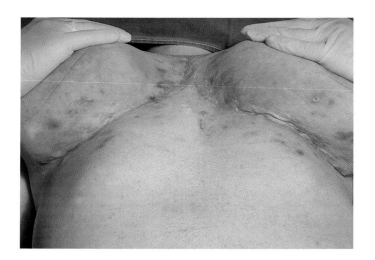

Figure 2.15a
Hidradenitis suppurativa/Inframammary area

This patient had a longstanding history of hidradenitis suppurativa. This disease of the apocrine glands is characterized by recurrent episodes of infection and draining abscesses. Pain, foul-smelling exudate, and inability to wear certain clothes, all contribute to a poor quality of life. Although mild cases tend to respond to systemic antibiotics, intralesional injections of corticosteroids, and good wound care, patients with established and active sinus tracts need a more aggressive therapeutic approach.

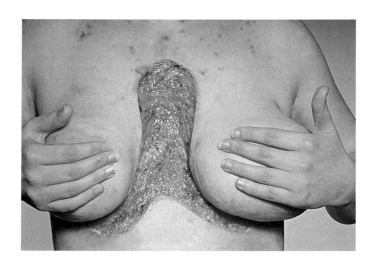

Figure 2.15b
Hidradenitis suppurativa/Inframammary area

The entire area was excised to remove all sinus tracts and tunneling. The patient healed well several months later. Also note the acneiform eruption on her chest. Patients often have both hidradenitis suppurativa and severe acne.

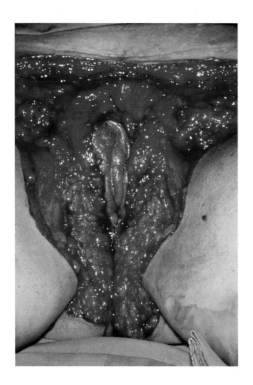

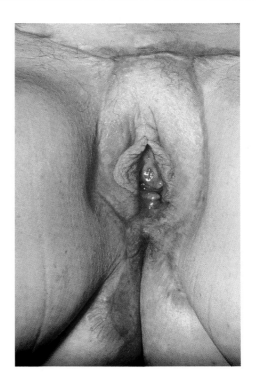

Figure 2.16a
Radical excision for hidradenitis suppurativa

This was obviously a patient with a very
extensive and severe case. There was no
choice but to remove the apocrine glands and
all of the sinus tracts that had formed over
the years.

Figure 2.16b
**Radical excision for hidradenitis
suppurativa/Follow-up**

Very acceptable result 3 months later.

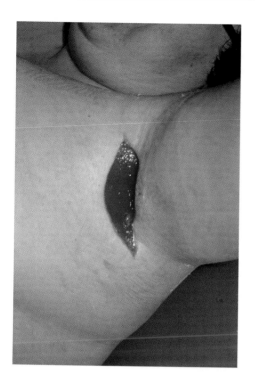

Figure 2.17
Excised area of hidradenitis suppurativa

This wound would not heal. In our experience, this type of livid red granulation tissue is actually not ideal and is frequently associated with infection or a heavy bacterial burden and may indicate local infection as a cause of non-healing.

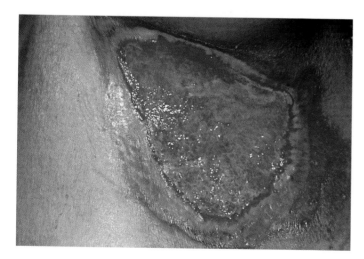

Figure 2.18
Wound after excision for hidradenitis suppurativa

In contrast to the previous case, the wound bed here may actually appear to be suboptimal. However, this particular wound shows evidence of healing and eventually healed completely. Apparent discrepancies between re-epithelialization and what we expect the wound bed to look like are not unusual. The general notion that granulation tissue in healing wounds should always be beefy red is probably an oversimplification. The red area lateral to the wound may represent a contact dermatitis.

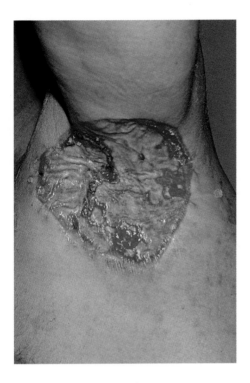

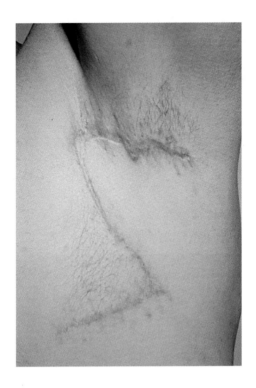

Figure 2.19
Excised wound of hidradenitis suppurativa/Grafting

Grafting is another way to deal with excised areas of hidradenitis. The rather thin graft in this case may act as both tissue replacement and a stimulus for wound repair. There seems to be some surface bacterial contamination of the wound bed, but the wound healed very satisfactorily.

Figure 2.20
Excised wound of hidradenitis suppurativa/Flap

This example of a z-plasty is shown to illustrate that there are a number of surgical approaches to the repair of wounds after excision of areas of hidradenitis. Here too the results are quite acceptable but unfortunately recurrence in the upper horizontal scar line shows the difficulty of obtaining cure by using primary closure.

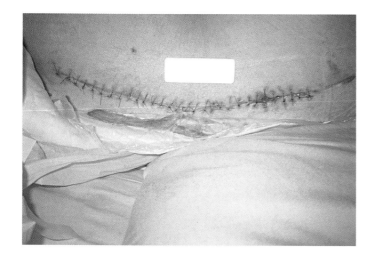

Figure 2.21
Sutured abdominal wound

This extensive wound was treated with dry non-adherent dressings. In our opinion, better cosmetic results are obtained by the use of semi-occlusive or occlusive dressings. However, there is still subtantial fear of using occlusion after such major surgical procedures. Many surgeons fear the development of infection and are concerned that the tensile strength of the wound does not develop normally in a moist environment. We believe that the fear of infection is generally unwarranted. However, further work needs to be done to study tensile strength of wounds treated by this method.

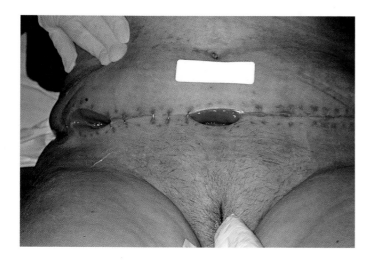

Figure 2.22a
Complication after urologic surgery

Here there was dehiscence of the surgical wound. By probing the two open wound areas we found them to be undermined and connected.

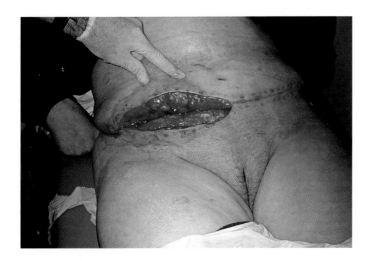

Figure 2.22b
Complications after urologic surgery/Clip removal

The clips over the skin bridge between the two open areas had to be removed. This then allows healing by secondary intention.

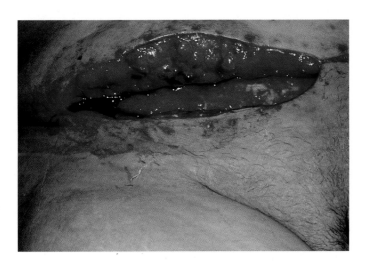

Figure 2.22c
Complications after urologic surgery/Close-up

This shows the early stage of healing before active granulation tissue has filled the whole wound area.

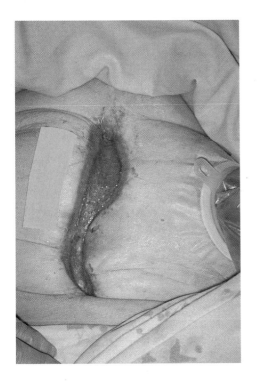

Figure 2.23
Healing wound after peritonitis

Surgery was required for treatment of a ruptured viscus and fecal peritonitis. The resultant wound shows a pink to red base and is healing well by secondary intention. Again, we would like to make the point that one should not expect a beefy red wound bed for optimal healing to occur.

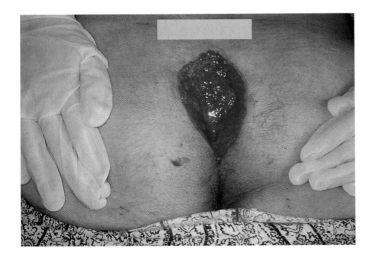

Figure 2.24
Pilonidal sinus surgery

These wounds will require several months to heal by secondary intention. Foam dressings or calcium alginates may be beneficial here to absorb the exudate. Some foam or hydrocolloid dressings from various manufacturers are specifically shaped for this area.

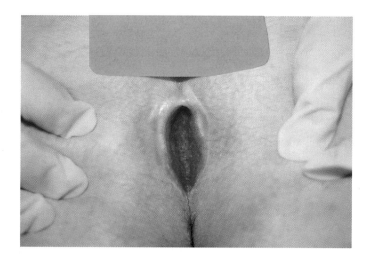

Figure 2.25
Pilonidal surgery

This wound resulting from excision of a pilonidal sinus did not heal completely, despite episodic decreases in the ulcer area. We have seen this happen before in patients with intragluteal ulcers. Whether the failure to heal is due to tension, faecal contamination, or pressure/friction, is unclear. Grafting may be a suitable alternative treatment.

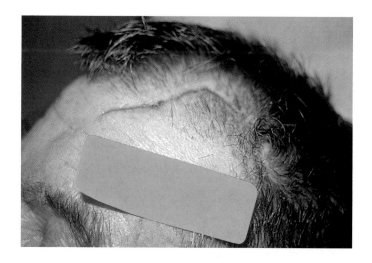

Figure 2.26
Sutured wound

This patient had a traumatic scalp laceration that required sutures. The photograph was taken immediately after suture removal. The redness can persist for many months, and often up to a year.

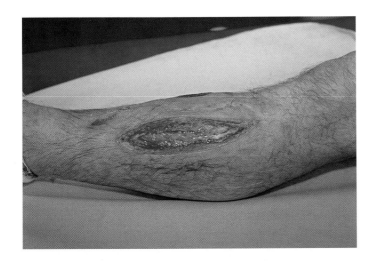

Figure 2.27
Open granulating wound

This excision became infected and a fasciotomy was necessary. The wound is now left open to heal by secondary intention.

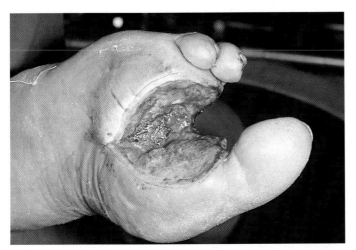

Figure 2.28
Granulating wound after amputation

This patient with diabetes mellitus required ray amputation of the second and third toes. The photograph shows the appearance of the granulating wound a week after surgery. One of the problems that will be encountered in this case is that other parts of the foot will now receive greater pressure during ambulation.

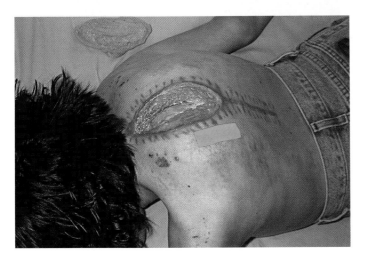

Figure 2.29
Complication of back surgery

This patient was referred after corrective surgery for spinal deformity. The large wound had been closed primarily. Unfortunately, the upper portion became infected and had to be opened to drain and heal by secondary intention. A foam dressing was used to absorb the considerable exudate. The development of osteomyelitis is a real concern here and it is probably better to let the wound heal secondarily.

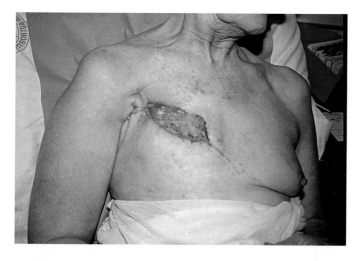

Figure 2.30
Grafting after mastectomy

Here too, after mastectomy, the wound became infected. However, a graft was eventually used to close the wound primarily. Most of the graft has taken and appears healthy.

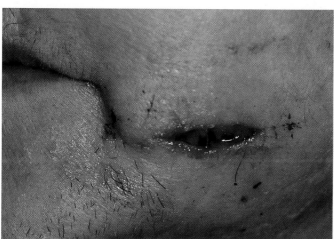

Figure 2.31
Wound dehiscence

This happens because of infection or excessive tension across the wound. In this case, wound dehiscence was due to infection. We prefer not to reclose these wounds primarily, and adherent strips or tape can be used to approximate the edges and still allow for drainage to occur.

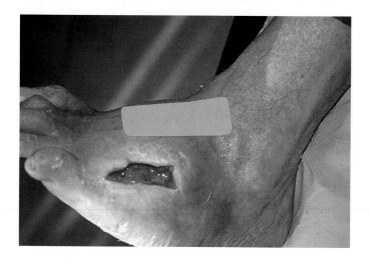

Figure 2.32
Abscess

After drainage of the abscess, the wound was left to heal by secondary intention. Calcium alginate dressings or foams would be useful in this situation because they are able to absorb a lot of exudate.

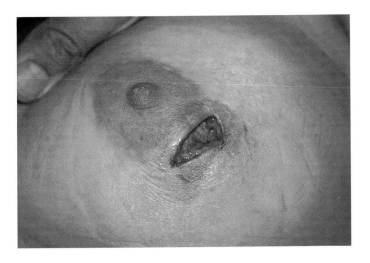

Figure 2.33
Breast abscess

A rather superficial infection eventually led to an abscess that needed to be drained. The photograph was taken after excision and drainage. Management of such a wound varies considerably among clinicians. Some still prefer the use of wet to dry dressings, while others might use calcium alginate material to absorb the exudate.

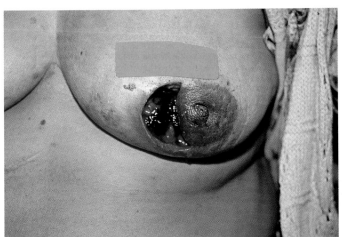

Figure 2.34
Hematoma after breast surgery

This large hematoma developed following surgery for duct ectasia. The clot needs to be removed and all bleeding vessels cauterized. A pressure bandage will be applied.

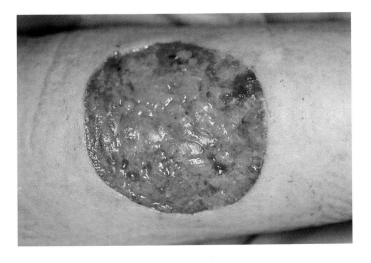

Figure 2.35a
Mohs wound and Graftskin

This woman in her fifties had a small papule on her right arm which, when biopsied, turned out to be a basal cell carcinoma. The extent of the tumor, removed by Mohs surgery, was surprising. At the end of the procedure, she was left with this very substantial full-thickness wound. Grafting with a full-thickness graft would be one way to approach this wound, given the risk of substantial contraction.

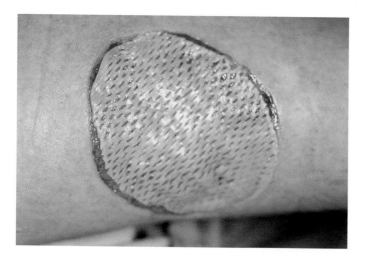

Figure 2.35b
Mohs wound and Graftskin/application

It was decided to treat this wound with Graftskin, a bioengineered skin product. Here one sees the wound covered with Graftskin, which was meshed at a ratio of 1.5 to 1. The pain improved immediately after the procedure. No sutures were used to hold the bioengineered skin in place, and the procedure was painless.

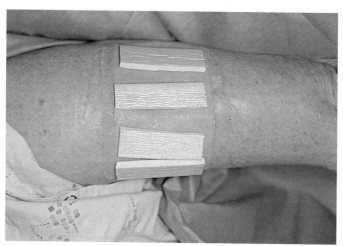

Figure 2.35c
Mohs wound and Graftskin/bolstering

We have found that a petrolatum-based gauze, also containing bismuth (Xeroform) can be ideal for dressing the wound after the application of bioengineered skin. As shown in the photograph, we place strips of a foam dressing over the primary Xeroform dressing. The purpose of the foam strips is to provide a bolster and still allow the escape of wound fluid.

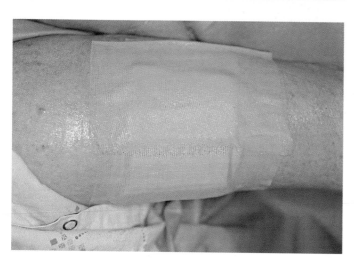

Figure 2.35d
Mohs wound and Graftskin/additional dressing

We basically create a 'foam dressing' with Xeroform (or similar dressing) on either side of the foam strips. The unit is remarkably stable and does not shift easily; generally, no sutures are required when using this type of graft coverage.

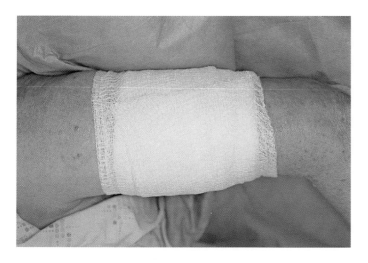

Figure 2.35e
**Mohs wound and
Graftskin/secondary dressing**

A gauze bandage is used to cover
the primary dressing. Often, we
follow this with a layer of self-
adherent elastic bandage. In our
experience, the dressing can stay in
place nicely for at least a week. Of
course, patients are told to be very
cautious in not disrupting the
dressing.

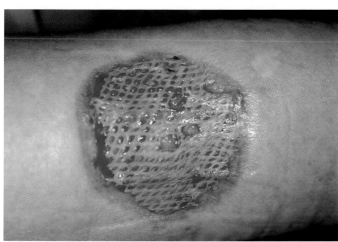

Figure 2.35f
**Mohs wound and
Graftskin/follow up at 1 week**

This was the appearance of the
wound 1 week after the
application of the bioengineered
skin. There seems to have been
good graft take, and one can easily
see the Graftskin in place over the
wound, which is now less deep. In
spite of the large size of this
wound, the patient did not
experience any pain.

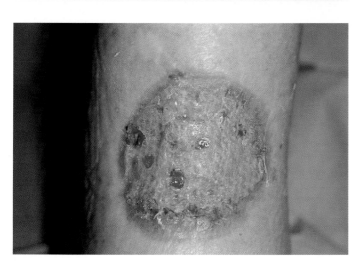

Figure 2.35g
**Mohs wound and
Graftskin/follow up at 3 weeks**

There has been remarkable healing
of the wound, no contraction, and
no pain. Moreover, because a
laboratory-grown, bioengineered
skin product was used, she did not
have a full-thickness donor site to
deal with.

3 Wounds and infection

Introduction

The diagnosis of infection in a wound is often obvious. One observes the cardinal signs of inflammation, the wound is not healing, and there may be systemic findings indicative of infection. However, the situation is not always clear-cut, especially in chronic wounds. Almost all chronic wounds are colonized with bacteria, many of them are surrounded by redness and are warm to the touch, and healing is often slow. Particularly in the elderly, who are unable to mount a substantial response to infection, wound pain and failure to heal may be the only signs that an infection is present.

There is still considerable controversy regarding the best way to diagnose infection. As mentioned, the mere presence of bacterial organisms within the wound is not sufficient. The clinical significance of redness and warmth surrounding the ulcer is often difficult to assess. Is it infection? Is it a contact dermatitis? Is it simply secondary to reflex vasodilatation, as occurs in arterial insufficiency? There have been attempts to arrive at the diagnosis of infection by obtaining a biopsy from the wound and by quantitating the number of organisms detectable in the tissue itself. This approach seems to be gaining acceptance, but a widely recognized scientific basis in support of its use, particularly for all types of wounds, is still lacking. Many clinicians feel that infection is a clinical diagnosis, and they tend to treat infection based on the appearance of the wound, the surrounding skin, the presence of certain organisms, systemic symptoms, and deterioration in the healing of the ulcer. There are other signs of infection that are not widely recognized but may be valid. For example, as shown by examples in this section, exuberant granulation tissue may signify infection rather than a good or excessive reparative response. Wound pain alone, as mentioned, may be a sign of infection.

In this section, we describe to a considerable extent the use of a slow-release iodine preparation to deal with excessive wound exudate and bacterial contamination of the wound. For years, iodine and other antiseptics were used to treat wounds, until it was realized in the early 1980s that some of these agents could interfere with the wound-healing process. However, the outcome was that clinicians basically stopped using antiseptics altogether. We feel that a considered approach to the use of antiseptics is of value in certain patients. Cadexomer iodine, a slow-release iodine preparation, may be very useful in the management of wound infection and colonization, particularly in highly exudative wounds. Other topical preparations may be useful as well, e.g. silver-based agents or dressings.

Bacterial infection is not the only one to complicate wounds. Astute clinicians must also think of more unusual infections. Particularly in the immunocompromised host, one must exclude infection with fungi, mycobacterial organisms, or even the presence of chronic infection with herpes simplex and cytomegalovirus. Rather than relying on swab cultures, one must often take biopsy samples to exclude these possibilities. Proper diagnosis demands that diagnostic material be taken immediately to the laboratory and be plated appropriately and under conditions which optimize the growth of fastidious organisms.

Wound debridement and systemic antibiotics are often necessary to deal with a significant wound infection. Hyperbaric oxygen therapy, combined with these approaches, is possibly useful as well. It is often believed that hyperbaric oxygen therapy is overutilized and that there is no definite proof of its efficacy. However, for deep infection (e.g. with anaerobic organisms), hyperbaric oxygen therapy may play a useful role. Systemic antibiotics alone are generally not effective unless they are combined with proper wound care and surgical debridement. Also, systemic antibiotics may not achieve appropriate concentrations at the wound site or may not be effective in the wound microenvironment (e.g. pH conditions, fibrosis).

Severe streptococcal infection remains a serious infection complicating wounds. The "flesh-eating bacteria" have received much attention. There is nothing to indicate that streptococcal infection and necrotizing fasciitis are on the rise. However, there are indications that, in addition to use of appropriate antibiotics and surgical approaches, the condition may benefit from systemic corticosteroids. At first, this may sound like a paradox, because systemic corticosteroids are often thought to predispose to or aggravate infection. However, the host response to infection may at times be a major problem, and systemic corticosteroids may help in dampening that damaging response. This approach remains controversial.

Clinical points

- The mere presence of bacteria in a wound does not signify infection.
- Infected wounds can be associated with a number of clinical findings, either together or by themselves: failure to heal, pain, necrotic tissue, local signs of inflammation, systemic symptoms and signs.
- The number of bacteria within tissue probably correlates with abnormalities in the way in which the host is dealing with invasion of microorganisms; the larger the number (i.e. greater than 10^6), the greater the possibility that the wound is infected.
- Occlusive dressings increase the number of microorganisms present in the wound fluid, but do not lead to infection.
- Exuberant granulation tissue, which at first may seem desirable, may actually represent infection.
- A translucent film over the wound tends to correlate with infection.
- Necrotic flaps may become infected, but with proper care and antibiotic therapy the tissue seems to recover and the results may be quite good.
- Not all antiseptics cause tissue injury. There are ways to deliver antiseptics in slow-release preparations; this helps keep the bacterial burden down.
- Surgical debridement is an excellent way to start treating infection in a wound.
- Hyperbaric oxygen therapy may be helpful in highly contaminated wounds.
- The only sign of necrotizing fasciitis is often exquisite tenderness, without any skin surface changes.
- Blistering around the wound may represent a contact dermatitis, but is also often seen with streptococcal infection.
- Blisters can also be caused by a staphylococcal toxin (as in staphylococcal scalded skin syndrome); this presentation is more common in patients with renal failure.
- Sharp demarcation of redness or blistering in the skin surrounding a wound can be seen with lymphangitis (erysipelas) and cannot be assumed to represent a contact dermatitis.

- The damage from streptococcal infection is often extensive and associated with a prolonged clinical course, in spite of antibiotic therapy. There is emerging evidence that in some cases systemic corticosteroids may be needed to decrease the host response to infection.
- Bites from brown recluse spiders can cause extensive necrosis and mimic a severe infection.
- Rapidly developing necrosis, especially on the extremities, should alert one to the possibility of meningococcal infection.
- Indolent necrotic ulcers, especially if present at multiple sites, may represent ecthyma gangrenosum, which is caused by bacteremias (commonly with *Pseudomonas aeruginosa*).
- When bone is exposed, it is fair to assume that it is infected (osteomyelitis).
- The development of puckering of the skin over an amputation stump may be associated with underlying bone collapse from osteomyelitis.
- Cellulitis not responding to antibiotics should alert one to the possibility of opportunistic infection, such as from cryptococcal organisms.
- The clinical appearance of the foot in leprosy may resemble that observed with the Charcot foot in diabetic patients. However, leprosy is associated with substantial resorption of bones.
- The use of a Wood's light may be helpful in the diagnosis of infection or colonization with *Pseudomonas* (green fluorescence) or corynebacteria (coral red fluorescence).
- Myasis (presence of maggots) is often missed. It should be suspected in all cases where an exudative dermatitis is present around the wound or involves the foot.

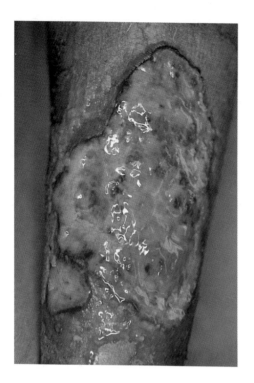

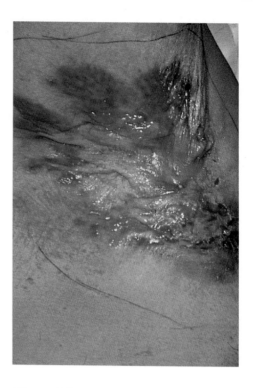

Figure 3.1
Heavily infeted ulcer

This venous ulcer is infected. The wound bed is purulent, necrotic, and appears to be heavily colonized with bacteria. The redness around the ulcer, particularly on the inferior border, suggests cellulitis. A biopsy from the wound bed showed acute inflammation and edema throughout the dermis and a deep abscess. Culture from the abscess grew both *Pseudomonas aeruginosa* and *Staphylococcus aureus*. The patient had to be hospitalized and required intravenous antibiotics and extensive debridement.

Figure 3.2
Hidradenitis suppurativa

The role of infection in this disease is not entirely clear, and often physicians treat these patients with intralesional injections of corticosteroids. In this case, the pain, tenderness, drainage and extent of the problem suggested that bacterial infection was present. She was treated with intravenous antibiotics. Eventually, extensive excision was necessary to control the disease.

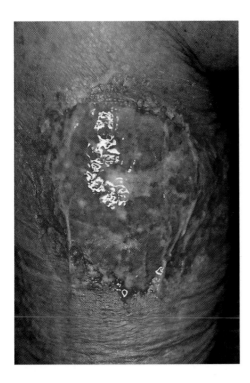

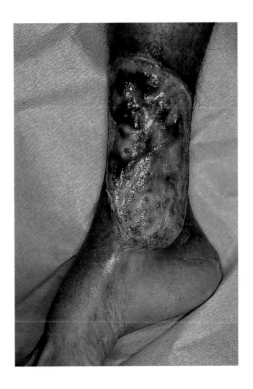

Figure 3.3
Infected tumor

This patient had cutaneous T-cell lymphoma. The skin tumor shown here ulcerated and became infected. The photograph shows a purulent wound seemingly covered by a film. Cultures from the wound grew *S. aureus*. She was treated with intravenous cephalosporins and the infection was controlled. When ulcerated, tumors frequently become infected.

Figure 3.4
Heavily colonized ulcer

This patient with sickle cell disease had a non-healing ulcer which was thought to be largely venous in etiology. However, it is likely that the underlying sickling plays a role in the pathogenesis and persistence of such wounds. The ulcer became heavily colonized with *P. aeruginosa*, requiring extensive debridement and antibiotic treatment.

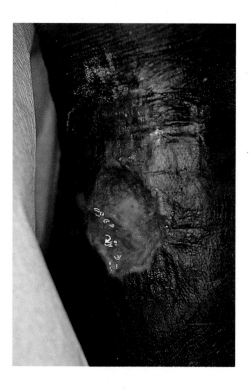

Figure 3.5
Infection in a recurrent ulcer

This venous ulcer on the lateral aspect of the ankle decreased in size by about 80% with compression bandages and dressings over almost a year. Eventually, the ulcer was grafted with an autologous split-thickness graft and the patient remained healed for 4 months. However, the ulcer recurred in the same location and is seen here at a time when it is infected. This clinical course is not uncommon in ulcers that are of long duration and are difficult to heal. It is essential that patients wear graduated stockings to help prevent recurrence.

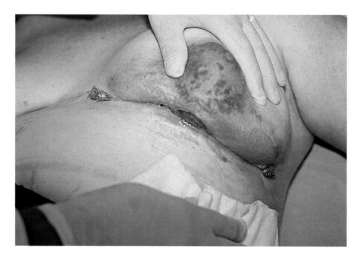

Figure 3.6
Infection after breast surgery

This patient had undergone surgery to her left breast but the primarily closed wound became infected. Here one can see the purulent exudate and the beginning of cellulitis in the surrounding skin.

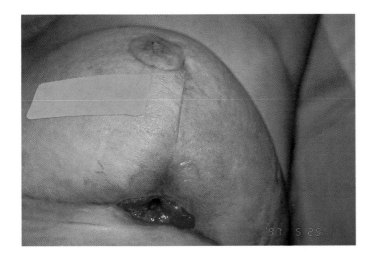

Figure 3.7
Abnormal granulation tissue

After a reduction mammoplasty, the suture line became infected. This granulation tissue looks abnormal in that it seems to extend over onto the surrounding skin, and it looks like a pyogenic granuloma. It may be necessary to remove this material and treat with antibiotics.

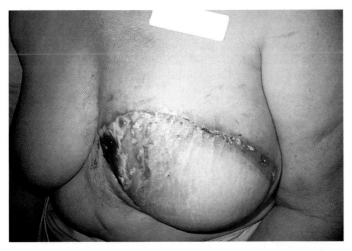

Figure 3.8
Breast infection and necrosis

Following mastectomy and breast reconstruction, the patient developed partial necrosis of the medial portion of the flap and cellulitis. Intravenous antibiotics and removal of the black necrotic tissue are necessary to manage this complication. Surprisingly, after controlling the infection, the results are often quite good despite suboptimal flap survival.

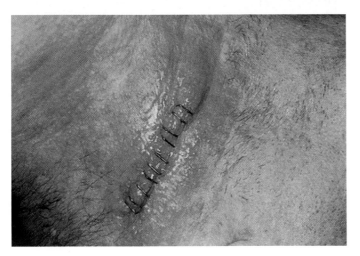

Figure 3.9
Contact dermatitis

Not all redness represents infection. Here the redness was due to the use of topical antibiotics, to which the patient was apparently allergic. The tiny vesicles around the wound are clues that this redness is more likely to represent contact dermatitis than a cellulitis. Pruritus, rather than pain or tenderness, is another useful clue pointing to contact sensitivity reaction. Sometimes, however, the distinction between cellulitis and contact dermatitis is impossible.

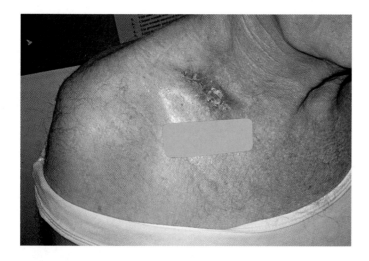

Figure 3.10
Infection in suture line

In contrast to the previous case, this patient had no pruritis but developed intense pain a few days after this wound in the supraclavicular fossa was closed primarily. The vesicular reaction observed in the previous case was not present here.

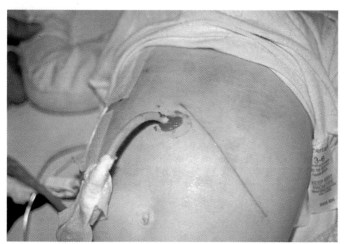

Figure 3.11
Excess granulation tissue

This child has a gastrostomy feeding tube. Many believe that excess granulation tissue, as seen here surrounding the orifice, represents infection. *S. aureus* is commonly found in such cases and should be the initial target of antimicrobial treatment.

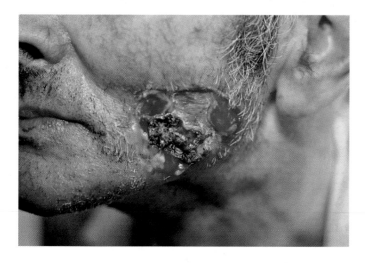

Figure 3.12
Graft failure

A skin graft was used to cover the defect after excision for a skin cancer. There is now partial failure of this graft, as shown by loss of graft take and necrosis. The reasons for this complication were not entirely clear, although infection may have played a role. Treatment requires removal of the necrotic portion of the graft and antibiotics.

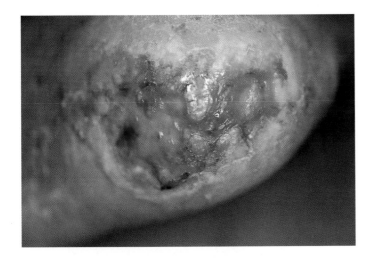

Figure 3.13
Graft infection

An autologous split-thickness graft was used to treat this heel ulcer due to radiation injury. The yellow color of the graft and the surrounding redness extending to the plantar surface point to the presence of infection. The graft will most likely fail, and one can already see uplifting of the graft posteriorly.

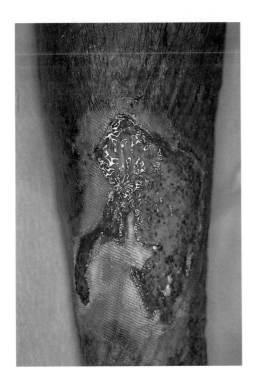

Figure 3.14a
Infected venous ulcer

This patient had a recurrent ulcer for 11 years and required frequent hospitalizations for cellulitis. For the past few weeks and months, the ulcer had been healing, as evidenced by the pink new skin devoid of pigment around the ulcer. However, at the time this photograph was taken, the wound bed had become purulent and showed the typical yellow fibrinous material suggestive of necrosis. As in other cases shown in this section, a translucent gelatinous film is covering the ulcer. We have seen this in many cases of infected ulcers. Cultures of this particular wound grew *P. aeruginosa*.

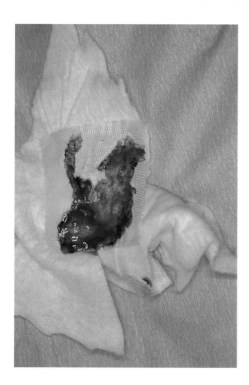

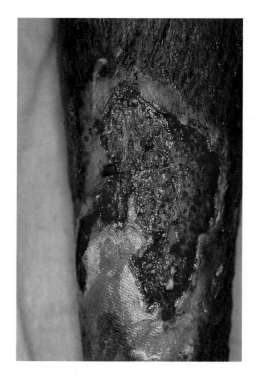

Figure 3.14b
Infected venous ulcer/Necrotic material

This photograph shows the exudate and necrotic material that came off with the removal of the dressings and compression bandage. The gelatinous film described in the previous legend is rather tenacious and stays on the wound. Mechanical debridement and whirlpool are potential ways of removing it.

Figure 3.14c
Infected venous ulcer/After whirlpool

This photograph was taken on the same day, immediately after one session of whirlpool. There is remarkable improvement in the appearance of the ulcer. The gelatinous film and much of the necrotic material are no longer present. A wedge biopsy was taken from the ulcer's edge for histology and microbiological studies. Contrary to what one might think, these biopsy sites heal extremely well, typically up to the original ulcer's margin.

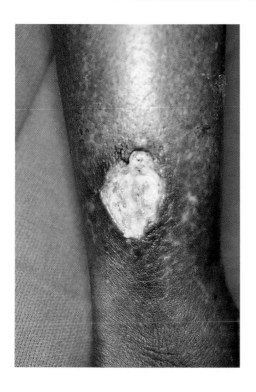

Figure 3.15a
Sickle cell ulcer

Leg ulcers in patients with sickle cell hemoglobinopathy are typically very painful and resistant to treatment. Their pathogenesis is not fully understood, but most likely involves abnormalities in both the venous and arteriolar circulation. As in this case, sickle cell ulcers are longstanding and frequently become infected or heavily colonized with bacteria.

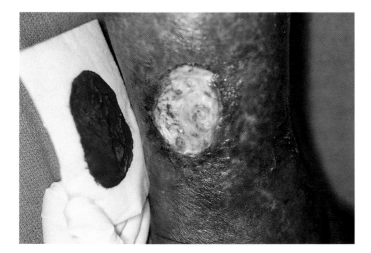

Figure 3.15b
Sickle cell ulcer/Cadexomer iodine dressing

Initial attempts at debridement in the outpatient setting were difficult because of severe pain. Cadexomer iodine is a good way to debride these ulcers and decrease the bacterial burden. Cadexomer iodine is a slow-release preparation of iodine that is non-toxic to chronic wounds. It is particularly helpful in large and exudative wounds.

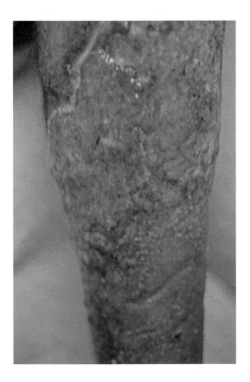

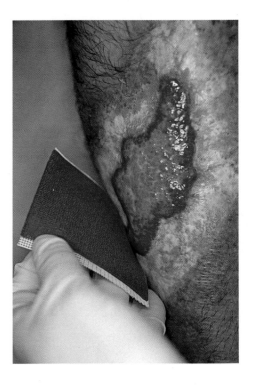

Figure 3.16a
Ulcers after bullous eruption

This 56-year-old man developed bullous lesions 1 day after receiving an IM injection of penicillin. Histology showed an intense neutrophilic infiltrate consistent with either Sweet's syndrome or pyoderma gangrenosum. Systemic work-up revealed a rare form of leukemia (chronic neutrophilic leukemia). He was treated with systemic corticosteroids and other systemic agents for the leukemia, and his course was complicated by non-healing ulcers on both legs. As seen in the photograph, poor granulation tissue and infection were a significant management problem.

Figure 3.16b
Ulcers after bullous eruption/Cadexomer iodine treatment

The patient's ulcers were treated with a hydrogel for the pain and, ultimately, with cadexomer iodine to debride the wound and decrease the bacterial burden. One of the organisms cultured from his ulcers was methicillin-resistant *S. aureus*. Although he was also treated in the hospital with intravenous antibiotics, we believe that a considerable reason for his improvement was the topical treatment with cadexomer iodine. The photograph shows that the ulcer has been healing and that there is now better granulation tissue. The white surrounding skin is due to hydration and maceration from the hydrogel. Cadexomer iodine is being re-applied to the wound.

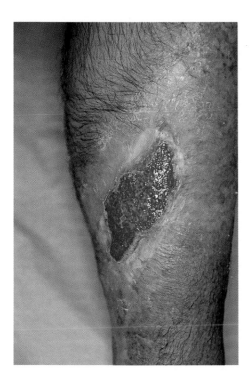

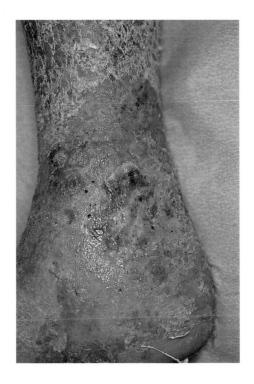

Figure 3.16c
Ulcers after bullous eruption/Follow-up

Local care with occlusion and with
cadexomer iodine seems to have decreased
the amount of yellow necrotic tissue in the
wound and the patient no longer required
mechanical debridement at each clinic visit.
New epithelium slowly migrated in from the
wound edges.

Figure 3.17a
Cadexomer iodine treatment

The patient has had recurrent and
longstanding venous ulcers. Contact
hypersensitivity to many topical agents has
further complicated his clinical course. At
this point, his ulcer is heavily contaminated
and is surrounded by severe dermatitis.
Patients with venous insufficiency have a
much greater incidence of sensitization to
topical agents and, in our opinion, should
avoid most topical treatments. Treatment
was initiated with surgical debridement and
compression bandages.

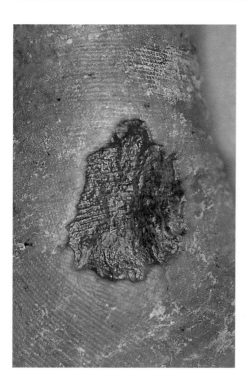

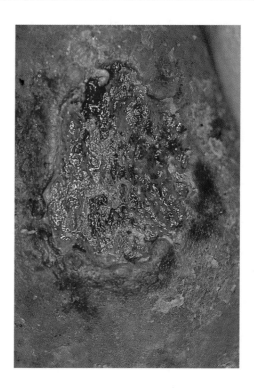

Figure 3.17b
Cadexomer iodine treatment/Follow-up

This picture was taken a couple of weeks later. The dermatitis has improved but the ulcer bed is still necrotic, particularly in the inferior portion. At this point, we made the decision to use cadexomer iodine.

Figure 3.17c
Cadexomer iodine treatment/Follow-up

This photograph was taken after another 2–3 weeks. The cadexomer iodine dressing has just been removed and one can see the residual orange–brown cadexomer iodine preparation around the edges of the ulcer. The ulcer bed now contains considerable epithelium and there is evidence of reepithelialization.

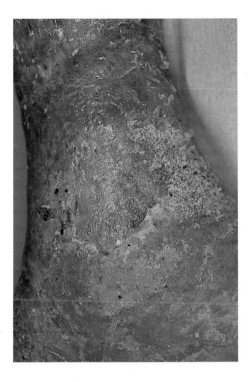

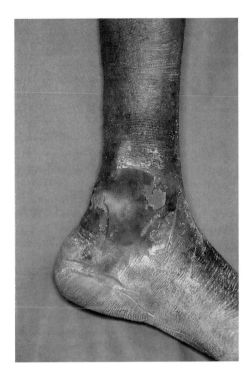

Figure 3.17d
Cadexomer iodine treatment/Follow-up

Six weeks later, the ulcer is virtually healed. The dermatitis is still present and will remain a management problem. We believe that many patients continue to use topical agents and thus perpetuate the dermatitis.

Figure 3.18
Cadexomer iodine gel/Before removal

There are two preparations of cadexomer iodine. The one shown here is a paste that is applied to a non-adherent pad and then placed on the wound. It is generally removed when the color changes from dark brown to an orange–yellow color, as seen here. The color change occurs within a couple of days, depending on the amount and quality of the exudate. Although the recommendation is to remove the cadexomer iodine at the stage shown in this photograph, we sometimes find it easier to change it daily. If possible, the material should be removed gently after soaking and without trauma to the wound.

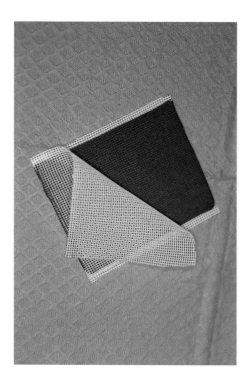

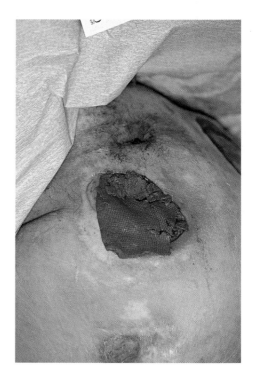

Figure 3.19a
Cadexomer iodine dressing

The other cadexomer iodine preparation is
the same gel but sandwiched between two
layers of a nylon mesh. This preparation is
often easier to use in deeper wounds.

Figure 3.19b
Cadexomer iodine dressing/Pressure ulcer

As shown here, the cadexomer iodine
dressing is used to dress these deep pressure
ulcers. Generally, the nylon layer in contact
with the wound is removed. Keeping the
outer layer during placement tends to
facilitate application of the cadexomer paste.
In this case, both sides of the dressing were
eventually removed.

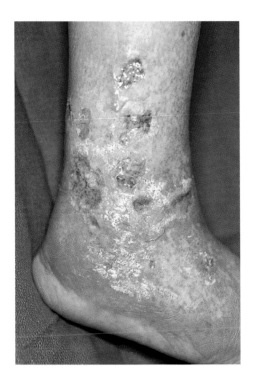

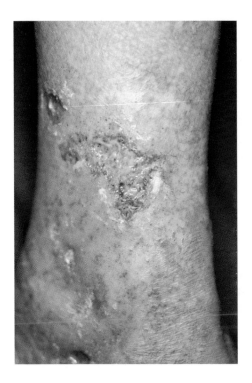

Figure 3.20a
Multiple ulcers

The etiology of these ulcerations was not
entirely clear. There are areas of atrophie
blanche and, histologically, fibrin thrombi
were present in the dermal vessels, suggesting
cyrofibrinogenemia or the antiphospholipid
syndrome. However, the major problem is
infection. These patients generally need to be
hospitalized for local care, whirlpool, and
intense treatment with antibiotics.

Figure 3.20b
Multiple ulcers/Close-up

The skin surrounding the ulcers is white and
studded with tiny blood vessels, a picture
typical of atrophie blanche. The term
atrophie blanche is purely descriptive and
does not tell us the etiology of the ulcers.
Atrophie blanche is seen not only in venous
and arterial disease, but also in vasculitis,
lividoid vasculitis, cyrofibrinogenemia, and
other conditions characterized by thrombosis
of cutaneous blood vessels.

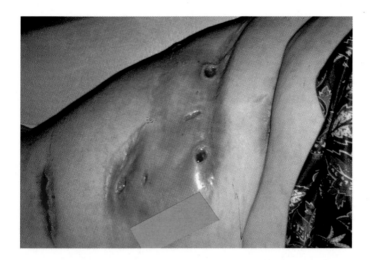

Figure 3.21a
Acute bacterial abscess

This very obese patient has had numerous abscesses in her right thigh. The area is tender and warm, and shows a lot of drainage.

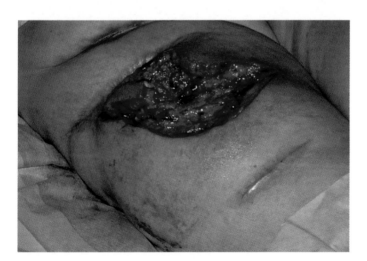

Figure 3.21b
Acute bacterial abscess/Follow-up

This photograph was taken after radical drainage of abscesses. Aggressive surgical debridement is necessary in such cases.

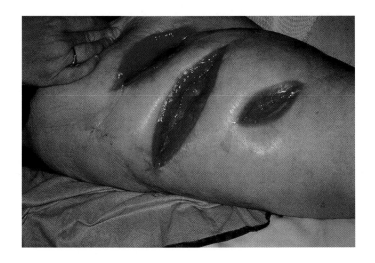

Figure 3.21c
Acute bacterial abscess/Follow-up

The same patient some weeks later. The wounds show good granulation tissue and are healing. Further surgical debridement has been necessary during her clinical course. Management is always difficult in these cases, and one has to be ready to perform multiple debridements.

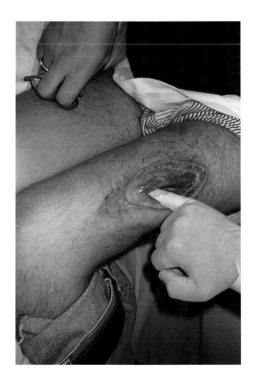

Figure 3.22
Bacterial abscess

Here too the abscess on this patient's thigh had to be opened and drained. As shown, there is extension to deeper tissues, which means that further debridement will need to be done.

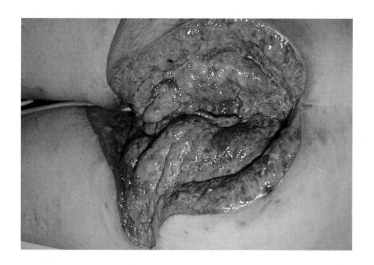

Figure 3.23
Perianal abscess

This photograph was taken following extensive surgery for an abscess in the perianal area in a patient with inflammatory bowel disease. The extent of debridement is dictated by the severity of the problem and tunneling to the subcutaneous tissues, and is best done in the operating room. Sometimes, these patients are also treated with hyperbaric oxygen.

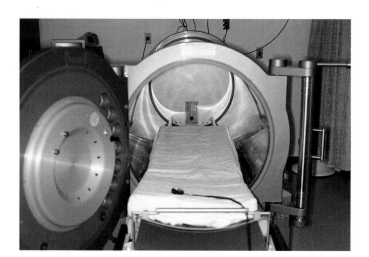

Figure 3.24
Hyperbaric oxygen chamber

This type of monoplace hyperbaric chamber can be found in many hospital settings. Hyperbaric oxygen is often used for difficult-to-heal wounds, particularly if they are heavily colonized. Although the evidence that hyperbaric oxygen is effective in treating wounds is not as good as one would like, there are situations where there seems to be a clear clinical benefit. Multiple treatments (i.e. 20 or more) lasting a couple of hours a day are often necessary.

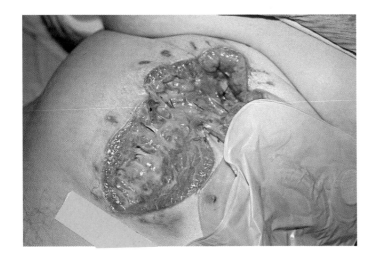

Figure 3.25
Complication of abdominal surgery

This woman has a large abdominal wound following emergency surgery for fecal peritonitis. There is healthy granulation tissue at the margins of the wound, but the wound bed shows suture material and proflavine-stained adipose tissue. It will take about 2 weeks to develop good granulation tissue throughout. Hyperbaric oxygen is occasionally used in this type of severe wound. One of the problems in evaluating the effectiveness of hyperbaric oxygen in chronic wounds is that this treatment is often reserved for the most complicated clinical situations.

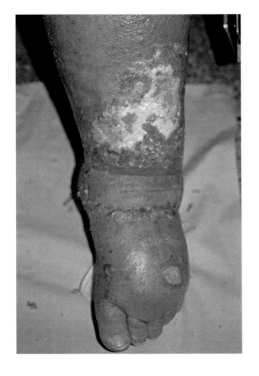

Figure 3.26
Leg swelling and cellulitis

There is little doubt that this patient has a severe cellulitis. The leg and foot are swollen, red, and weeping. The entire lower leg was warm to the touch. Systemic symptoms of fever and chills were present. This is a life-threatening condition and needs to be treated on an emergency basis with hospitalization and intravenous broad-spectrum antibiotics. Recently there have been reports that systemic corticosteroids should be used in addition to the antibiotics. However, this has not become standard practice yet.

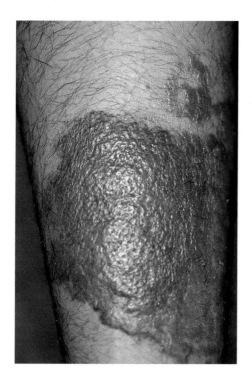

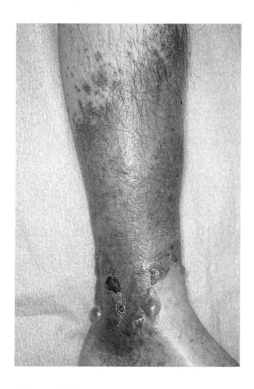

Figure 3.27
Cellulitis

This purpuric eruption was thought to
represent a vasculitis, but there was fever and
no histologic evidence of vasculitis. He
eventually responded to intravenous
antibiotics. We have seen this type of
presentation rarely, but believe that it may
represent a streptococcal infection
(erysipelas). It points to the need for careful
clinical and pathologic correlation.

Figure 3.28
Cellulitis with blisters

The patient responded to intravenous
antibiotics. Cultures were negative, but one
would strongly suspect that this condition is
due to streptococcal infection. This illustrates
the difficulty of identifying the causative
organism in all cases of such infection.

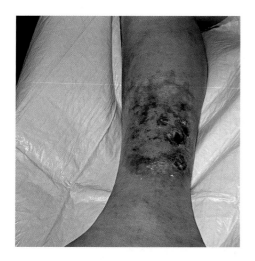

Figure 3.29
Unusual cellulitis

This patient was thought to have a cellulitis, but it took almost 3 weeks of intravenous antibiotics for her to improve. Brown recluse spider bite would be in the differential diagnosis, as would vasculitis. Histology, however, did not show vasculitis.

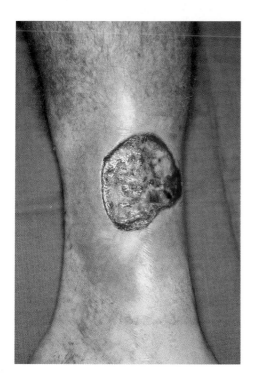

Figure 3.30
Cellulitis

The appearance of the wound is not always indicative of whether it would cause a severe infection. Here the ulcer itself does not look very colonized or infected, but the redness and warmth around the wound indicate a cellulitis.

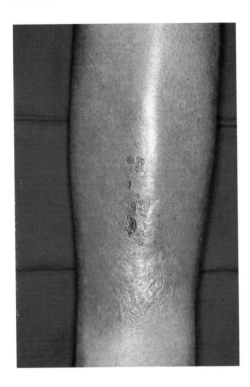

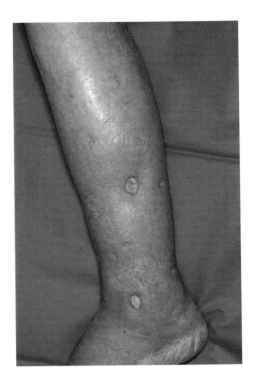

Figure 3.31
Cellulitis and lymphedema

This 72-year-old woman has lymphedema.
The clinical clue is that the leg is "tubular"
in appearance and does not show the typical
exaggerated narrowing towards the ankle
that one sees in venous disease. Because of
the lymphedema, she suffers from repeated
bouts of cellulitis which require
hospitalization. The skin was warm and red.
Usually, no systemic symptoms or
leucocytosis were present, but the absence of
these signs is common in the elderly with
infection. She was eventually managed with
the use of long-term oral penicillin therapy.

Figure 3.32
Cellulitis and punched-out ulcers

The presence of cellulitis is rather obvious
here. The warm and red skin extends from
the foot to the mid-portion of the leg. She
also had severe arterial insufficiency.

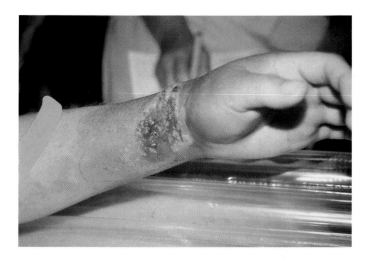

Figure 3.33
Extravasation of cytotoxic drugs

He had severe soft tissue damage at the intravenous site on his forearm following extravasation of chemotherapeutic drugs. Adriamycin and 5-fluorouracil are particularly toxic agents that can cause this. The inflammatory response is probably not due to infection, but often such patients are treated with systemic antibiotics.

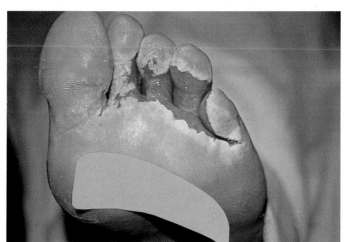

Figure 3.34
Streptococcal infection

The skin is denuded and there is considerable maceration. The patient had a streptococcal infection.

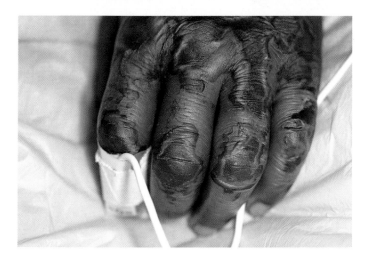

Figure 3.35
Meningococcemia

This life-threatening infection can cause massive necrosis within hours. This 28-year-old man presented to the emergency room in shock and was immediately admitted to the intensive care unit. Many of the fingers and toes became necrotic and began to ulcerate. Debridement was needed to manage some of these necrotic areas. He survived after a prolonged hospital course.

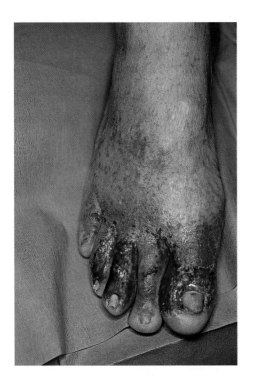

Figure 3.36
Infection and maceration

This man has venous disease of his leg and foot. The purpura and swelling of his toes is associated with infection. He was treated with systemic antibiotics and whirlpool. In these cases, it is difficult to apply compression bandages without making the problem worse, because the toes may become even more swollen with leg compression.

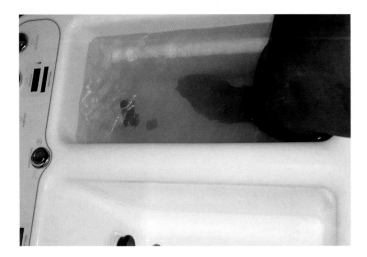

Figure 3.37
Whirlpool treatment

There is considerable controversy still as to whether whirlpool treatment helps in the debridement and healing of ulcers. We have found it helpful in certain situations (e.g. draining wounds) and have used it in combination with surgical debridement and antibiotic therapy. In some cases, our patients come in and have a whirlpool session once or twice a week after dressing removal and before the application of a new dressing.

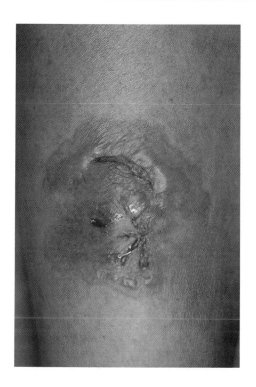

Figure 3.38
Recurrent erythema multiforme

Not all infections are due to bacterial organisms. This 34-year-old woman has lesions on her lower legs that begin as red spots, enlarge, and form a central blister. Hydrogel dressings have been used to decrease the intense pain present within these lesions. Many cases of recurrent erythema multiforme are now recognized to be a complication of infection with herpes simplex. She is being managed with the systemic administration of acyclovir, dapsone, and occasional courses of systemic corticosteroids.

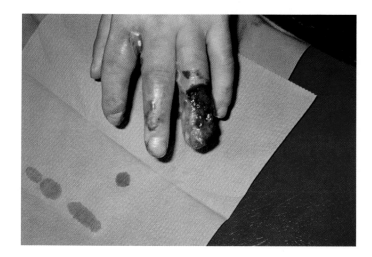

Figure 3.39
Skin fragility in Ehlers–Danlos syndrome

These disorders are characterized by features of hyperextensible skin and joint hypermobility. In patients with Ehlers–Danlos type II (autosomal dominant inheritance), skin fragility can be a problem and can lead to spontaneous ulceration and necrosis, as shown in this photograph. Debridement and antibiotics will be necessary in this patient. Hyperbaric oxygen will also be an option. One has to be sure that there is no underlying osteomyelitis.

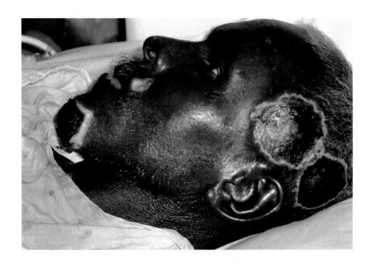

Figure 3.40
Ecthyma gangrenosum

This man with leukemia has septicemia and has developed these dark ulcerated lesions of ecthyma gangrenosum. This entity is usually due to infection with *Pseumonas aeruginosa*, but can also be seen with other types of bacteria. The occurrence of this infection portends a very poor prognosis.

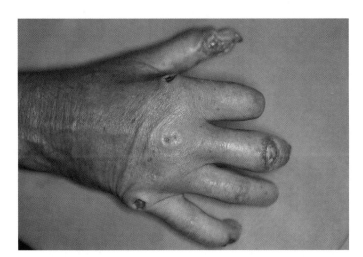

Figure 3.41
Scleroderma ulcers

Patients with systemic sclerosis (scleroderma) commonly develop hand and finger ulcerations. The ulcers on the tips of the fingers, as seen here, are probably due to a fixed vascular narrowing and do not readily respond to vasodilators. Ulcers on the knuckles are usually precipitated and perpetuated by trauma. Occlusive dressings can help in the painless debridement of these ulcers.

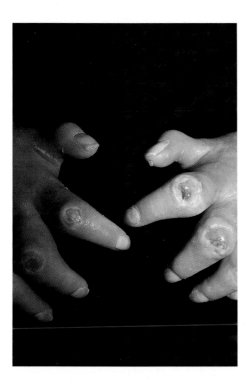

Figure 3.42a
Scleroderma ulcers and septic arthritis

This patient with systemic sclerosis (scleroderma) had longstanding and non-healing ulcers on her hands. Eventually, she developed septic arthritis in the involved joints. Although this occurrence is not common, we want to stress the point that there is a tendency to underestimate the possibility of serious infection in patients with scleroderma ulcers.

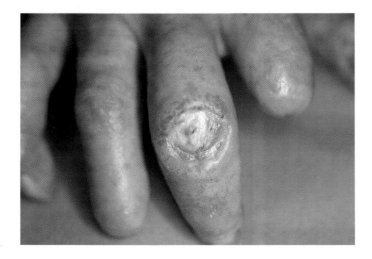

Figure 3.42b
Scleroderma ulcers and septic arthritis/Close-up

The bone is partly exposed. It is said that osteomyelitis is usually present when one can actually see or touch the underlying bone.

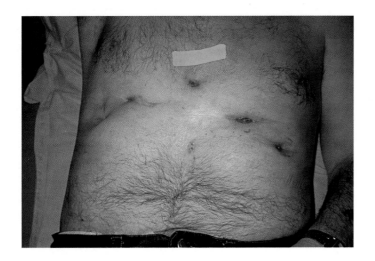

Figure 3.43
Osteomyelitis from septicemia

This is an unusual case where the patient became septic following a flare-up of inflammatory bowel disease. Osteomyelitis subsequently developed along the whole of the margin of his lower ribs. The photograph shows five separate wounds due to sinus tracts. When multiple wounds are present, one should be aware of the possibility of a systemic process and septicemia.

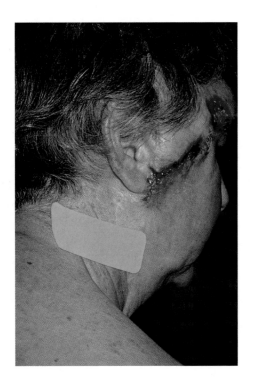

Figure 3.44
Osteomyelitis of the face

The possibility of osteomyelitis should always be considered in situations where healing is delayed. This woman had multiple surgical procedures for an extracranial tumor and required skin and bone grafting. She did not heal, and there was continued drainage at the wound site. Eventually, she was found to have osteomyelitis of the bone graft.

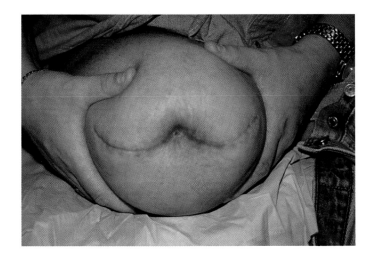

Figure 3.45
Osteomyelitis in a stump

Sometimes, the presence of osteomyelitis is totally unexpected. In this man with an above-knee amputation, there were no obvious clinical signs of skin infection except for puckering of the skin and some crusting. However, there was failure to heal and further studies showed underlying osteomyelitis due to methicillin-resistant *S. aureus*. The skin puckering is due to underlying bone collapse. Further amputation was required.

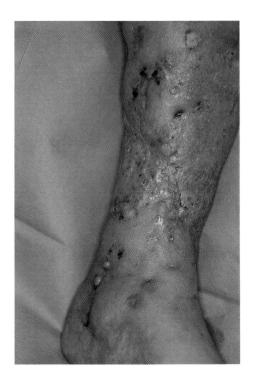

Figure 3.46
Mycobacterium ulcerans

There are multiple small ulcerations and draining sinuses. Some areas look healed, while others appear to be necrotic. There has been considerable scarring, suggesting a prolonged clinical course. *Mycobacterium ulcerans* grew from cultures of skin tissue. She was treated with a combination of clofazamine, clarithromycin, and trimethoprim/sulfamethoxazole. Surprisingly, she was not immunocompromised.

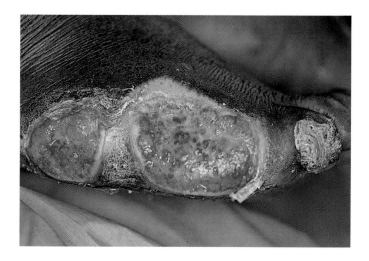

Figure 3.47
Atypical mycobacterium infection

There was no clear explanation for this man's bilateral foot ulcers and their failure to heal. He had these for about 8 months. The seemingly good granulation tissue and re-epithelialization at the edges of the wounds probably delayed the diagnosis. Multiple bacterial cultures showed a variety of organisms and he did not respond to standard antibiotic treatment. Tissue taken from the wound, however, grew an atypical mycobacterium, and the ulcers responded to intravenous amikacin. The patient had diabetes mellitus, but there was no other known cause for immunosuppression.

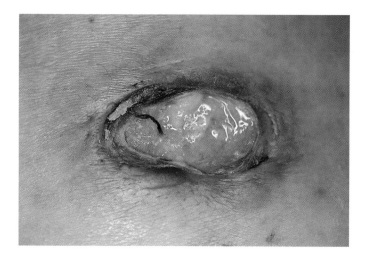

Figure 3.48
Disseminated mycobacterial infection

This woman with chronic myelogenous leukemia developed septicemia and this non-healing ulcer. She did not respond to usual wound care. Eventually, tissue from the ulcer grew an atypical mycobacterium that was resistant to multiple antibiotics. Dramatic improvement occurred with kanamycin, biaxin, and interferon therapy.

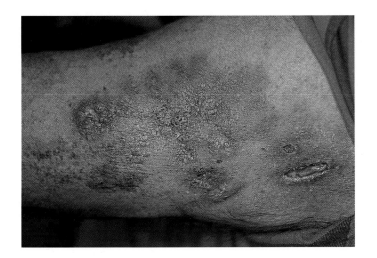

Figure 3.49a
Mycobacterium infection and immunosuppression

This patient was immunocompromised from the use of long-term systemic corticosteroids and methotrexate for psoriasis. Initially, this eruption on his left upper arm looked like a folliculitis and was treated with oral antibiotics. However, he did not respond to this treatment and actually developed multiple abscesses on his left upper arm and leg. The photograph mainly shows nodules and ulcers. Culture of tissues from these areas grew *Mycobacterium fortuitum*.

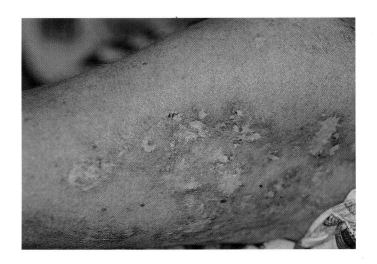

Figure 3.49b
Mycobacterium infection and immunosuppression/Healed ulcers

An indwelling catheter was used to deliver antibiotics intravenously for over a year. His infection resolved, although considerable scarring is present.

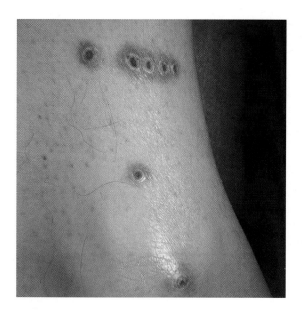

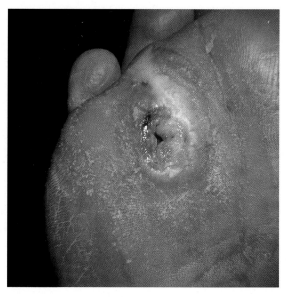

Figure 3.50
Aspergillus infection

These pustules distributed in a linear pattern were found to be due to aspergillus infection. The patient had received a liver and pancreas transplant and was on intense immuno-suppressive therapy. He responded quite well to systemic antifungal therapy. One must always be alert to the possibility of unusual infections in immunocompromised patients.

Figure 3.51
Neuropathic ulcer from leprosy

At first, this foot ulcer looks very much like what one might see in patients with diabetes mellitus and neuropathy. However, in this case the neuropathy was due to Hanson's disease (leprosy). The ulcer is very deep and the patient will require extensive surgical debridement.

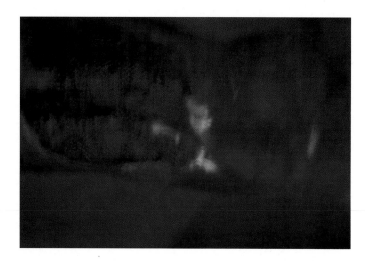

Figure 3.52
Wood's lamp examination

The coral fluorescence seen here with a Wood's light suggests infection with a corynobacterium. The Wood's light can be helpful in identifying gross infection with certain organisms, including *Pseudomonas aeruginosa* (green fluorescence).

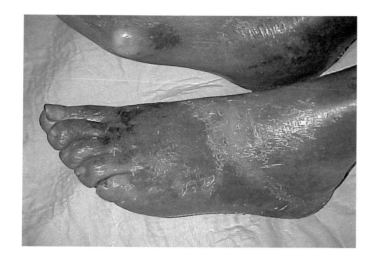

Figure 3.53a
Venous ulcers complicated by myasis

This elderly woman with venous ulcers was being cared for by her sister at home. She was hospitalized because of cellulitis. There was considerable maceration in the interdigital spaces of her feet. Tiny worm-like insects (maggots) were seen in that location.

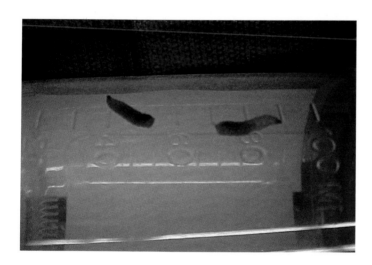

Figure 3.53b
Venous ulcers complicated by myasis/Larval forms

This photograph shows maggots found in her wounds. The patient did very well with whirlpool and intravenous antibiotics, and was discharged after a few days. Although there has been a revival of the use of maggotts for the purpose of debriding wounds, it is unlikely that this therapy will become popular again. The maggots do not actually eat or suck tissues, but secrete fluid containing a number of proteolytic enzymes that are able to break down only necrotic tissues. However, maggots also affect keratin, and so non-ulcerated skin is also damaged by these insects.

4 Pressure and neuropathy

Introduction

The injury caused by simple pressure is often underestimated, both in terms of the time required for tissue necrosis to develop and for the extent of necrosis to become apparent. It is good to keep in mind that pressure injury leads to ulcers characterized by deep tissue necrosis and loss of volume that are disproportionately greater than the overlying skin defect. Therefore, the area of ulceration may be misleading and will tend to lead to underestimation of the true extent of the problem. There is a well-described pressure-induced "cone of injury" with its base towards the underlying bone. This might explain the skin undermining which characterizes pressure ulcers; the skin is less susceptible to injury than the underlying tissues. Muscle and other subcutaneous tissues are highly susceptible to pressure injury because of direct or shearing forces on large segmental and perforator arteries; it has been argued that skin necrosis from pressure is less likely because the cutaneous blood supply benefits from nearby anastomozing vessels. This is only one explanation for why skin and subcutaneous tissues differ in their susceptibility to pressure. For example, in experimental animal models, degeneration of muscle fibers and full-thickness skin necrosis occur after 60 mmHg for 1 h and 600 mmHg over 11 h of contact pressure, respectively. As clinicians are well aware, the anatomic location of pressure is also an important variable, as pressures over 2500 mmHg are reached immediately over bony prominences. Also, it appears that patients with neurologic or vascular abnormalities, e.g. diabetes or spinal cord injury, are more susceptible to pressure injury.

As in diabetes, many ulcers due to pressure are thought to result from loss of protective sensory input. The neuropathy of diabetes leads to many structural changes in the foot. Extensor function is altered, and this causes excessive prominence of the metatarsal heads. Autonomic failure is likely to play a pathogenic role as well. Thus, there is decreased sweating and more easily damaged skin. However, whether the "insensate foot" alone fully explains the development of ulceration remains somewhat unclear. There are a host of abnormalities (metabolic, vascular, neurologic) in patients with diabetes, and these deficits are likely to play a fundamental role in creating the conditions leading to pressure injury and ulceration. For example, patients with diabetes have long been thought to have "small vessel disease". The role of this abnormality in the development of pressure injury is unclear. We do know that an obstructive vascular lesion of small blood vessels is unlikely. We also know that there are structural and functional abnormalities of the endothelium and blood vessels in patients with diabetes, e.g. excessive thickness of the basement membrane, endoneural capillary damage, and vascular leakage of albumin and other proteins. Hyperviscosity and fibrin deposition are also described. In addition to neuropathy, patients with diabetes suffer from increased susceptibility to vascular abnormalities, including atherosclerosis and medial sclerosis. Because of this, many clinicians now believe that the ankle to brachial pressure index (ABI), which is often used to exclude severe arterial insufficiency, is not useful and is often unreliable in patients with diabetes.

Throughout this section, we describe clinical cases where control of infection is a critical component of care in patients with pressure (decubitus) or diabetic ulcers. Extensive surgical debridement removes infected and necrotic tissue and stimulates the healing process. Debridement should remove the undermined edges of the ulcer, because these areas act as a pocket for bacterial growth. Also, in patients with neuropathic diabetic ulcers, one should remove the callus surrounding the ulcer. This process of "saucerization" creates a wound that has flatter edges and contains healthier tissue. In this regard, a popular notion is that aggressive surgical debridement transforms a chronic wound into an "acute wound". This may be partly true, but it is probably too simplistic. As further explained in this section, removal of tissue from within and around the wound may actually be removing cells that have been adversely altered by the long-standing pathogenic events (i.e. pressure and ischemia). Bringing new young cells in may provide the wound with healthier and more active cells, at least for a period of time. We discuss this further in the section on vascular ulcers.

The metabolic abnormalities associated with diabetes (e.g. impaired migration of neutrophils and macrophages) do seem to predispose to infection. From the practical standpoint, it is important to achieve maximal glucose control. It is also worthwhile to try and correct clinical abnormalities that might lead to infection. For example, although this has not been studied in detail, it is probably important to treat tinea pedis and onychomycosis in patients with diabetes. By decreasing skin dryness and fissures associated with fungal infection, one might also decrease the chance of bacterial entry and infection. Certainly, this approach is worth pursuing in patients with recurrent cellulitis.

Clinical points

- Diabetic ulcers can develop as a result of ill-fitting shoes and from sharp objects which end up inside shoes. Patients with diabetes should always shake their shoes before wearing them.
- Treatment of tinea pedis and onychomycosis may help patients with diabetic ulcers by preventing the development of cracks in the skin and bacterial entry leading to cellulitis.
- Off-loading is essential to ulcer care in diabetic patients. The notion of the insensate foot is generally poorly understood by patients and requires continuous reinforcement.
- Total contact casting is a useful first approach in the management of Charcot foot.
- The area of ulcers in pressury injury is often misleading; there is often a deeper component that is not immediately obvious.
- Pressure ulcers in the heel are often complicated by vascular problems.
- Exposed bone generally means osteomyelitis.
- Proper debridement of diabetic ulcers should include complete removal of the surrounding callus.
- Because they may provide an ideal pocket for infection, the undermined edges of pressure ulcers should be removed surgically.
- Especially in the elderly, hip fracture and hospitalization are major risk factors for pressure ulcers.
- Measurements of pressure ulcers require that volume be assessed. An easy way is the use of alginate material to obtain a mold of the ulcer.
- Because of non-compressible or only partly compressible arteries, the ABI in patients with diabetes does not reliably exclude arterial insufficiency.

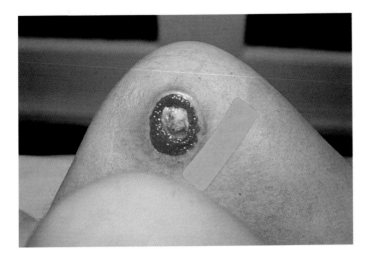

Figure 4.1
Pressure ulcer in a paraplegic patient

Such ulcers on the medial aspect of knees are not uncommon in patients with spinal cord injury and spastic paralysis. In this case, there was rather constant trauma to the medial aspects of both knees. Although much of the ulcer has excellent granulation tissue, the center is necrotic and in need of debridement. Management of these ulcers involves the use of protective dressings, such as hydrocolloids, or foam padding.

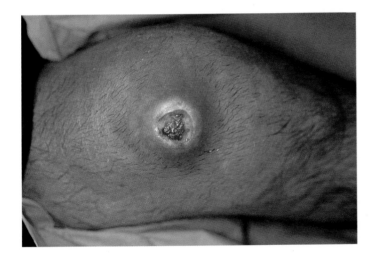

Figure 4.2
Pressure ulcer from trauma

This patient, too, was paraplegic. In his case, he could only sleep comfortably in a prone position. However, spasm caused continuous trauma to the knee and led to the development of this ulceration. There is substantial callus formation around the ulcer. Again, clinical management requires medications to decrease spasm, soft mattresses, and foam padding. Hydrocolloids or foam dressings are helpful in wound debridement, protection, and absorption of exudate.

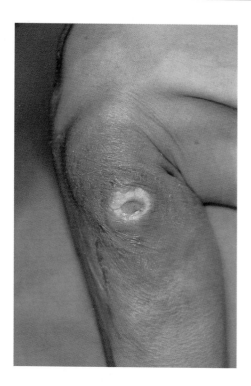

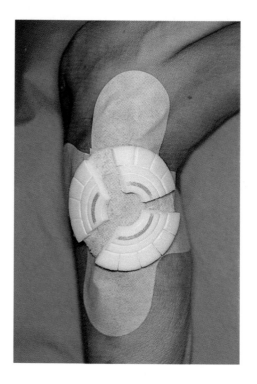

Figure 4.3a
Pressure ulcer in a patient with multiple sclerosis

As in the two previous cases, this woman suffered from a severe neurologic deficit and sustained pressure injury to her knee. Her course was also complicated by the development of eosinophilia myalgia syndrome secondary to the ingestion of L-tryptophan.

Figure 4.3b
Pressure ulcer in a patient with multiple sclerosis/Wound dressing

This special pressure relief dressing, which combines a hydrocolloid with foam rings on top, can be modified and cut to accommodate the contour of the area to be treated. It seems to work best in situations such as this, where intermittent trauma and not constant pressure is the problem.

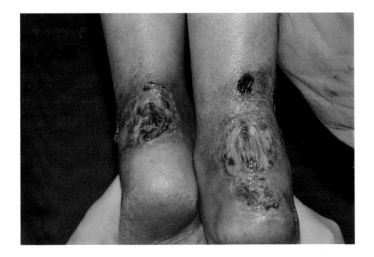

Figure 4.4
Pressure injury to the back of the ankle

This patient was from a nursing home and had stage IV pressure ulcers. She also had severe arterial insufficiency. Although this is an extreme case, it does highlight the need to monitor patients with neurologic deficits for the development of ulcers in any areas of pressure. For example, we have seen pressure ulcers developing on the calf of diabetic patients undergoing hemodialysis in a recliner for several hours at a time. The extent of the ulcers in this particular case makes management very difficult. Most likely, the Achilles tendons will have to be cut and the entire area debrided extensively.

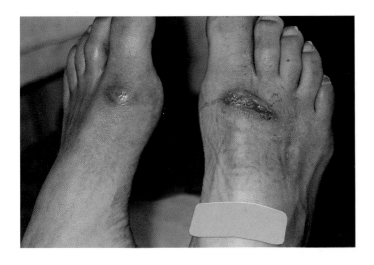

Figure 4.5a
Pressure ulcers from ill-fitting shoes

In diabetic patients with severe neuropathy, ulcers do not develop only at the bottom of the foot and toes. In this case, the shoes were the culprit, and this woman developed ulcers at pressure points on the dorsal aspect of her feet.

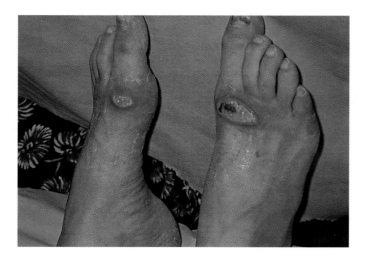

Figure 4.5b
Pressure ulcers from ill-fitting shoes/Follow-up

Unrelieved pressure caused the ulcers to worsen. Patients such as this one need to have custom-made shoes. Made-to-fit sandals can be used until custom shoes are ready. Also note the scaly rash in a moccasin distribution, especially evident on the left foot. This and the appearance of the nails strongly suggest dermatophyte infection, which was confirmed by potassium hydroxide examination and cultures. Newer systemic agents are highly effective for treating fungal infections and should be used in these patients, because infection and cellulitis commonly occur from skin cracks developing as a result of the infection. Dermatophyte infection in a moccasin distribution does not respond well to topical antifungal agents

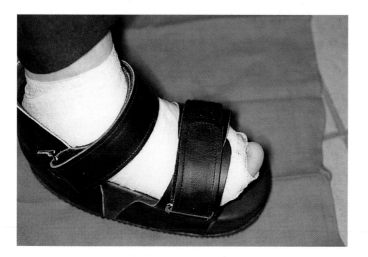

Figure 4.6a
Healing sandal

There are many varieties of sandals and shoes for patients with diabetes or other neuropathies. The one shown here is commonly used and is made to fit, after taking an impression of the patient's sole.

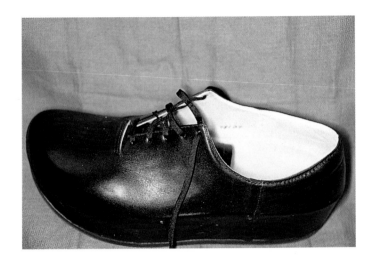

Figure 4.6b
Custom-made shoe

Patients with neuropathic ulcers have to be fitted for such shoes by specialized personnel. Often, it takes several weeks for the shoes to be ready. Although custom-made shoes are expensive, they appear to be a worthwhile and cost-effective means of preventing further ulcers. Conversely, poorly made shoes or changes in weight distribution can actually cause ulcers. Clinicians and the patient need to monitor this closely.

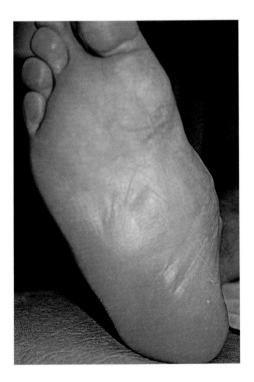

Figure 4.7
Charcot foot

Neuropathic changes and still poorly understood factors leading to alterations in the alignment of the bones in the foot may cause fracture dislocations and severe inflammatory reactions. Here, the bulging on the medial aspect of the midfoot is due to this process. Conservative treatment with total off-loading or, possibly, with total contact casting is the first and best approach. The use of systemic anti-inflammatory agents is still controversial. Ulcers commonly develop when the foot has changed shape to such a degree.

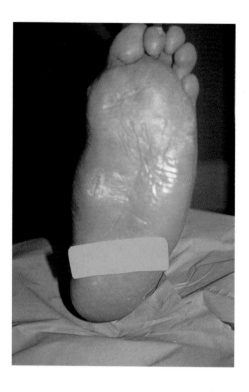

Figure 4.8
Charcot foot with ulceration

The gross deformities present in this foot are chronic and in time may require both medical and surgical intervention to prevent recurrent ulcers. An ulcer on the first metatarsal head has healed but is still very much susceptible to recurrence. Again, proper custom-made shoes and off-loading are essential.

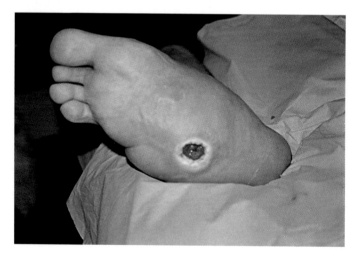

Figure 4.9
Charcot foot and deep ulceration

Another example of what can happen when the bony structures of the foot become more prominent and cause sustained pressure from walking or standing. The ulcer is surrounded by a large callus which needs to be debrided and saucerized for maximal ulcer healing. The white portion of the callus around the ulcer is due to hydrated skin. We have found that patients with neuropathy, such as this one, need continued education and reinforcement about the relationship between pressure and ulceration. We have been impressed by the fact that this rather simple concept is not fully understood by many individuals.

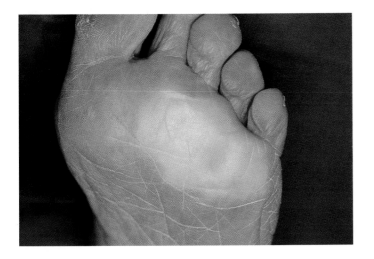

Figure 4.10
The effect of pressure on blood flow

Pressure causes very substantial decreases in local blood flow, and this photograph is a vivid demonstration of this. A glass slide was placed for a few seconds against this elderly woman's sole. Although not much pressure was applied, blanching of the skin is quite evident. One can extrapolate this finding to the situation encountered by patients with diabetes or other neuropathies. These patients unknowingly place sustained pressure on their feet and, as a consequence, develop prolonged ischemia and necrosis. The technique shown here can be used as a teaching tool to show patients how pressure compromises blood flow.

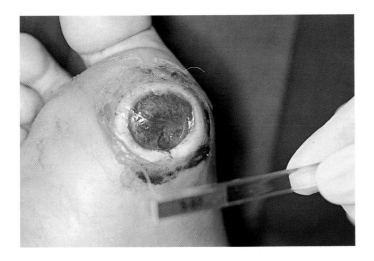

Figure 4.11
Large neuropathic ulcer

This young man with diabetes developed this ulcer about 9 months ago. The ulcer is surrounded by an extensive and thick callus. He has complete loss of sensation in his feet. Application of a Weinstein filament, seen here at 7 o'clock, does not elicit any sensation. Treatment of the ulcer requires extensive debridement of the callus and saucerization of the wound.

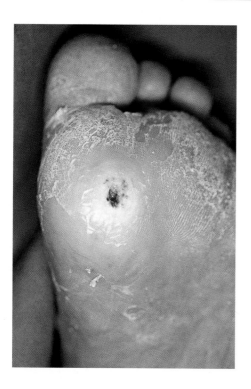

Figure 4.12a
Diabetic neuropathic ulcer

It is easy to underestimate the actual size and depth of ulcers in patients with pressure injury. Here the ulcer appears to be rather small and surrounded by a callus. However, pressure injury has been shown to affect the subcutaneous tissues more than the skin. Therefore, there is often a cone of injury with the base of the cone in the deeper tissues.

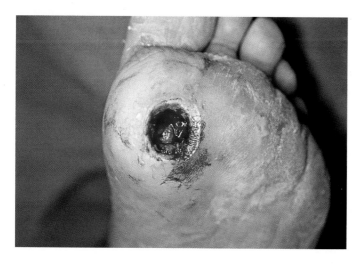

Figure 4.12b
Diabetic neuropathic ulcer/Debridement

Using a scalpel, the callus was removed and the debridement carried out down to bleeding and healthy tissue. The difference in susceptibility to injury between skin and subcutaneous tissues also explains undermining; the overlying skin is less affected while the tissues beneath it become necrotic.

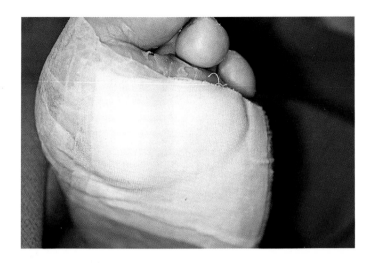

Figure 4.12c
**Diabetic neuropathic
ulcer/Debridement**

A pressure dressing was applied
right after the debridement and
kept in place for a few hours.
However, one must be careful that
off-loading is carried out, or else
the additional padding from the
dressing could exacerbate the
extent of pressure injury to the
site. The use of topically applied
platelet-derived growth factor
(Regranex) has been shown to
accelerate the healing of these
ulcers.

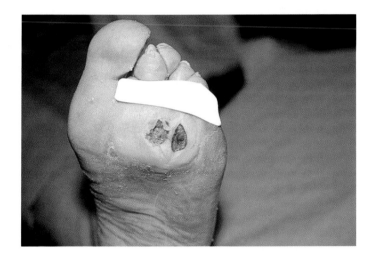

Figure 4.13
Large callus and ulcer formation

Here the amount of pressure has
been substantial, and the clinical
appearance cannot really be used
to assess the amount of necrosis of
the underlying tissues. For
management, one needs to remove
this entire callus and debride
down to the subcutaneous tissues
and bone. It is quite possible that
osteomyelitis is present at this
stage.

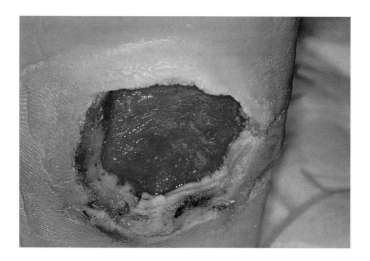

Figure 4.14
Diabetic ulcer with good granulation tissue

Some clinicians might be content with the way this neuropathic ulcer looks, because of the good granulation tissue in the ulcer base. However, we strongly advise removing the surrounding callus for optimal ulcer healing. The presence of callus generally implies poor compliance with off-loading. There are, however, some cases where we have observed continued callus formation despite immobilization and proper off-loading. Studies are needed to evaluate this phenomenon and whether it might represent chronic alterations in the cellular phenotype of the skin.

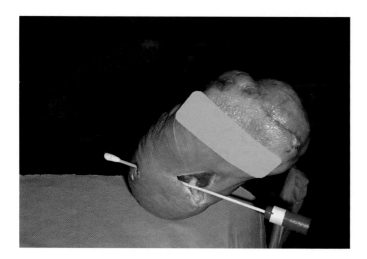

Figure 4.15
Sinus tract in a neuropathic ulcer

One needs to be aware of the possibility that ulcers might be communicating through sinus tracts, as illustrated here. The presence of these subcutaneous tunnels alters management dramatically, and this complication requires extensive debridement. The patient has previously lost his toes because of pressure injury.

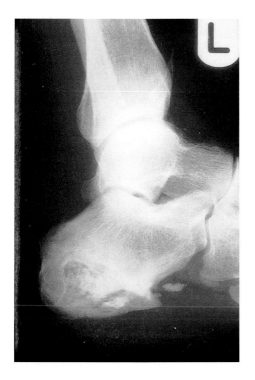

Figure 4.16
Osteomyelitis of the calcaneous

The heel is commonly affected by pressure injury, and ulcerations occurring in this area are frequently complicated by vascular problems and osteomyelitis. Therefore, one should not think of heel ulcers as simply being secondary to neuropathy. In this case, radiographic examination confirmed the presence of osteomyelitis.

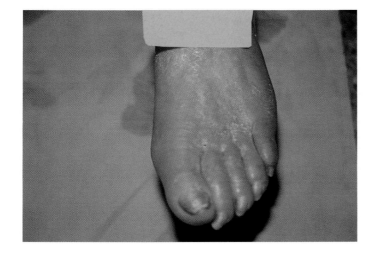

Figure 4.17
Arterial insufficiency in diabetes

The red appearance of the foot may suggest cellulitis. However, it is not uncommon for the redness to be due to arterial insufficiency alone. There is also extensive fungal infection. Maceration between the toes is also a problem here, and is due to edema of the toes and poor blood supply. This patient may require systemic antibiotics and antifungal agents, whirlpool treatment, and cautious separation of the toes with cotton material. He was being evaluated for arterial bypass.

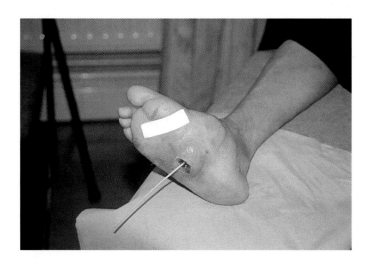

Figure 4.18
Deep neuropathic ulcer

Once again, it is often surprising how deep some of these ulcers are. Bone could be touched here with the cotton-tipped probe. It has been shown that osteomyelitis is present once bone is exposed.

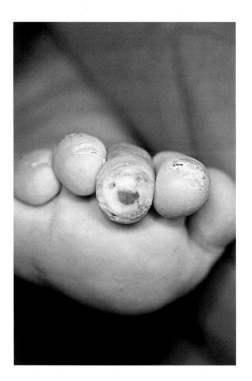

Figure 4.19
Pressure ulcer on the third toe

This patient with longstanding diabetes and peripheral neuropathy has had this pressure ulcer from a hammer toe deformity for several months. The ulcer goes through periods of partial healing and enlargement. Ideally, one should remove the surrounding callus and have the patient evaluated for correction of the hammer toe. One should realize that it is important to warn patients that, while debridement is necessary, it will create a much larger ulcer. Topical platelet-derived growth factor (Regranex) would be a good therapeutic option here.

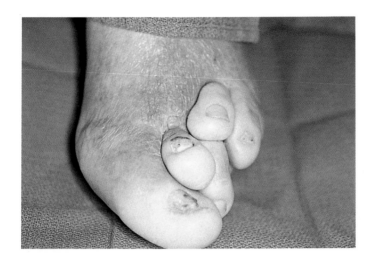

Figure 4.20
Diabetic foot after multiple surgical procedures

This patient had several operations to remove metatarsal bones. The toes were not removed, however. This is a mistake, because the non-functional toes merely create a situation where pressure from the shoes or within the toes leads to further ulcerations.

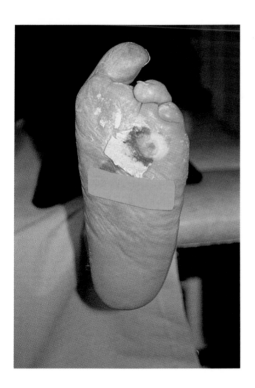

Figure 4.21
Exudative diabetic ulcer

Neuropathic ulcers in the diabetic patient are often not very exudative. In this case, however, the considerable drainage necessitated the use of an absorbant dressing, such as an alginate. Alginates are capable of absorbing large amounts of wound fluid. There is still some controversy over whether diabetic ulcers should be occluded, but most clinicians appreciate that moist wound healing accelerates healing and leads to painless debridement.

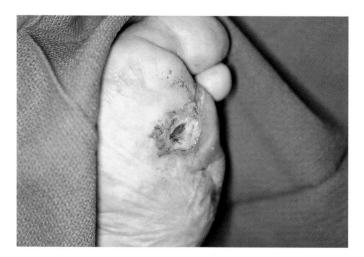

Figure 4.22a
Diabetic ulcer treated with a living skin equivalent

This man had recurrent ulcers on the metatarsal heads. Here the ulcer is surrounded by callus that needs to be removed.

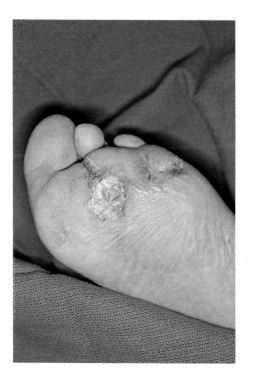

Figure 4.22b
Diabetic ulcer treated with a living skin equivalent/Follow-up

After debridement, the skin equivalent was applied to the ulcer. This living skin equivalent is bilayered and made up of human keratinocytes and dermal fibroblasts derived from neonatal foreskin. The fibroblasts are embedded in a type I bovine collagen matrix. Slits are often made in the living skin equivalent, so as to allow the escape of exudate from the wound, or else the "graft" would be uplifted. Overlapping of the living skin equivalent onto the wound edges seems to increase its adherence and prevent it from shifting.

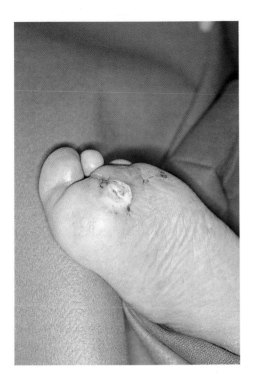

Figure 4.22c
Diabetic ulcer treated with a living skin equivalent

This photograph was taken 3 days after the application of the living skin equivalent. There appears to be actual take.

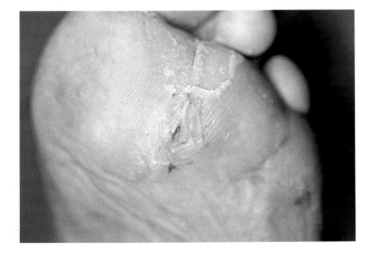

Figure 4.22d
Diabetic ulcer treated with a living skin equivalent

Complete healing of the ulcer occurred within 2 weeks. At this point, there is no exudate appearing on the dressing. We could not be sure as to whether the living skin equivalent remained on the wound or whether it provided a stimulus for wound repair. Tissue engineering technology and its application to the treatment of wounds has emphasized that grafts act not only as replacement, but also as cell therapy, capable of delivering growth factors and other stimulatory substances.

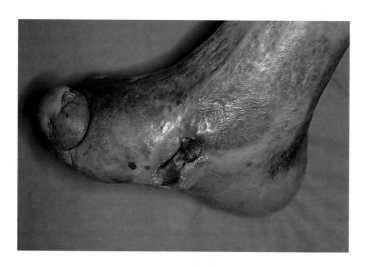

Figure 4.23
Patient with leprosy

The neuropathy in this patient was secondary to Hansen's disease (leprosy). The ulcer is due to pressure because of the insensate foot. While at first this clinical picture may resemble the ulcers due to diabetes, in fact resorption of the toes is more typical of Hansen's disease.

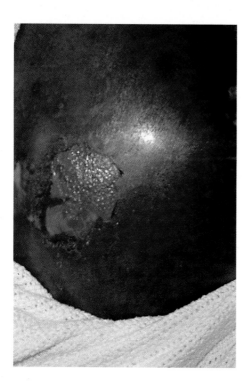

Figure 4.24
Stage II pressure ulcer

There is partial-thickness skin loss on the hip involving epidermis, dermis, or both. The ulcer is superficial and presents clinically as an abrasion, blister, or shallow crater. The photograph was taken in a hospitalized patient who was unable to shift position in bed. Removal of pressure, proper positioning in bed, flotation mattress and use of protective dressings (i.e. a hydrocolloid), are measures that could be used to treat this condition and prevent it from worsening.

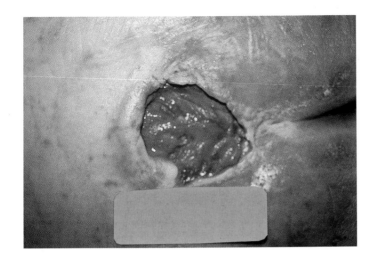

Figure 4.25
Stage III pressure ulcer

There is healthy granulation tissue in the base of this sacral ulcer, which extends down to the subcutaneous tissues. There is undermining, which is quite typical of pressure ulcers because of the increased susceptibility of deeper tissues to pressure injury, compared to skin. The redness around the ulcer may represent the early stages of pressure injury (stage I). Thorough debridement of the ulcer and undermined portions need to be done. Indeed, bacterial overgrowth often develops under the undermined edges.

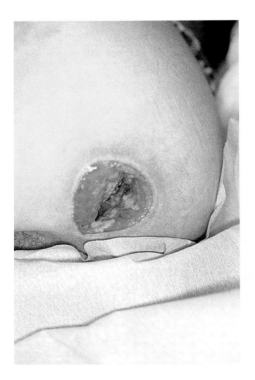

Figure 4.26
Stage IV pressure ulcer

This young girl of 7 was in an automobile accident and became paraplegic. The ulcer developed from prolonged pressure as she spends most of the day in a wheelchair. Pressure relief devices placed over the seat of the chair did not help. The ulcer extends down to bone. When faced with such ulcers, it is best to excise all of the necrotic tissue and bone in the operating room.

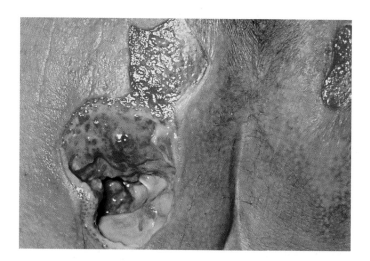

Figure 4.27
Multi-stage pressure ulcers

These sacral pressure ulcers are in different stages of development, from non-blanching erythema (stage I), to partial-thickness skin loss (stage II), to extension into the subcutaneous tissue (stage III), and bone involvement (stage IV).

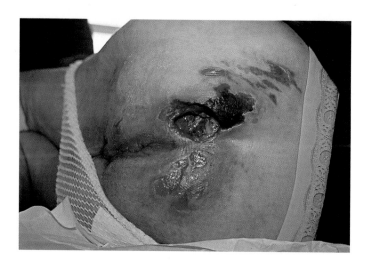

Figure 4.28
Multi-stage pressure ulcers

Some of these are necrotic and covered by an eschar, while others below show some evidence of re-epithelialization. The blisters above the necrotic sacral ulcer may be secondary to friction injury. The development of pressure ulcers, besides immobility, is often due to friction and incontinence. Especially in the elderly, hip fracture and hospitalization often lead to pressure ulcers.

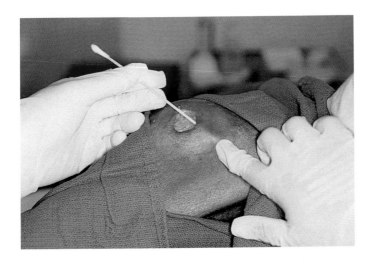

Figure 4.29
Undermining of pressure ulcer

The extent of undermining in pressure ulcers can be considerable. Here the wooden probe can be inserted several centimeters away from the ulcer. Unless one probes these ulcers, the extent of damage to the subcutaneous tissues is underestimated. Most clinicians advise removing all skin overlying the undermined areas.

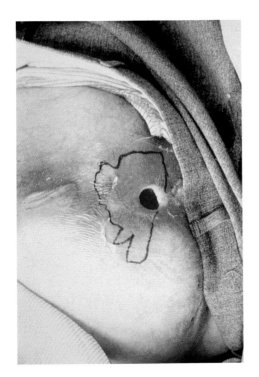

Figure 4.30
Undermining of ischial ulcer

Here the area of undermining has been traced over the skin. This area was subsequently completely excised and the resultant cavity packed with saline-soaked gauze although alginate or hydrogel packing could also have been used.

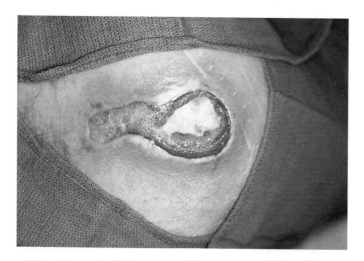

Figure 4.31a
Pressure ulcer over a hip prosthesis

This had been a recurrent ulcer. The white area was immediately over the prosthesis.

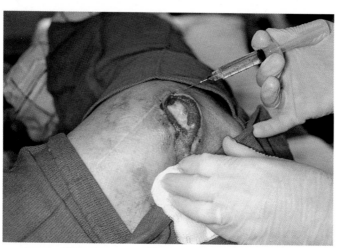

Figure 4.31b
Pressure ulcer over a hip prosthesis/Debridement

The area was first anesthetized with 2% lidocaine with epinephrine. Besides helping in pain control, the preparation also diminishes bleeding during the debridement.

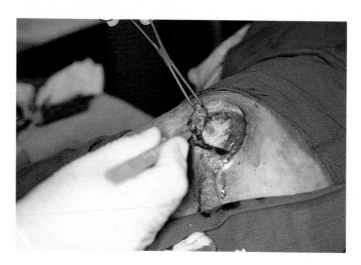

Figure 4.31c
Pressure ulcer over a hip prosthesis/Debridement

Extensive debridement with a scalpel and scissors showed the ulcer to be much larger and deeper than initially assessed.

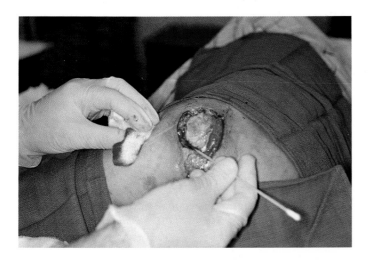

Figure 4.31d
Pressure ulcer over a hip prosthesis/Debridement

Probing of the edges is always a useful maneuver to judge the extent of deep tissue injury. This is often done repeatedly during debridement, to be sure of removing all necrotic and undermined tissues.

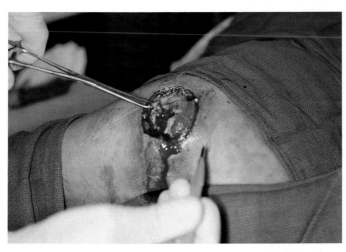

Figure 4.31e
Pressure ulcer of a hip prosthesis/Debridement

Further debridement over the center of the ulcer showed that the hip prosthesis was directly exposed. The patient had to be taken to the operating room to have the hip prosthesis removed.

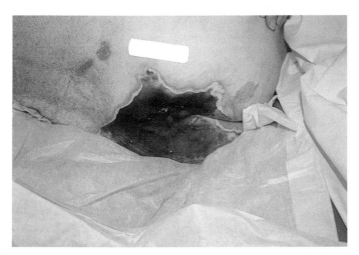

Figure 4.32a
Massive necrosis due to pressure

This large sacral ulcer in a nursing home patient needs immediate attention to remove the eschar and drain any possible underlying abscess.

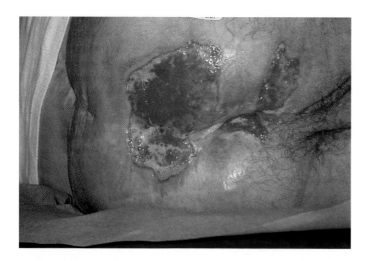

Figure 4.32b
Massive necrosis due to pressure

The same ulcer 2 weeks later, after debridement and nursing attention to relieve the pressure. This patient has a good chance to heal. Portions of the wound bed are yellow and still necrotic, and could probably use additional debridement. This could be achieved surgically or with autolytic debridement with a hydrocolloid or hydrogel.

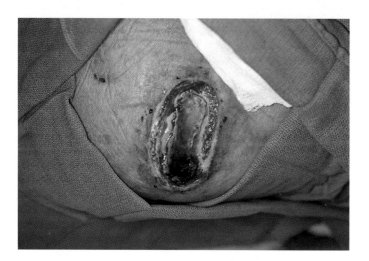

Figure 4.33a
Debridement and measurements of pressure ulcers

This patient with multiple sclerosis had a stage IV pressure ulcer on his hip. The eschar within the wound must be removed to a healthy bed.

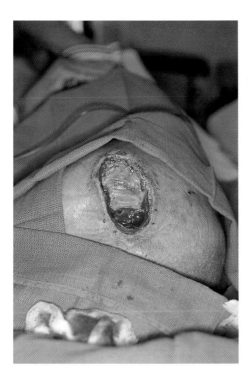

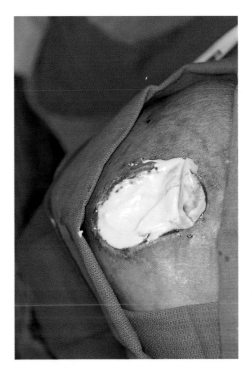

Figure 4.33b
Debridement and measurements of pressure ulcers

The eschar was removed, and the wound bed still showed fibrinous material which required further debridement.

Figure 4.33c
Debridement and measurements of pressure ulcers

This dental alginate material has commonly been used to obtain an impression and a volume measurement for deep wounds, such as pressure ulcers. The material, consisting of a powder, is mixed with water and then applied in its semiliquid form into the wound. Occasionally, it is helpful to cover the wound first with a film dressing, and then apply the alginate solution through a slit in the film and using a large-bore syringe. The alginate solidifies quickly. It can then be easily removed from the wound and weighed to obtain an objective measurement of wound size.

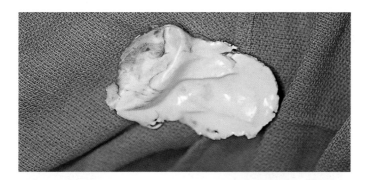

Figure 4.33d
Debridement and measurements of pressure ulcers

The alginate mold soon after removal from the patient's ulcer.

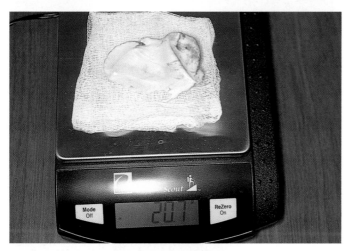

Figure 4.33e
Debridement and measurements of pressure ulcers

The alginate mold being weighed. The weight can be used to objectively assess the progress of the ulcer.

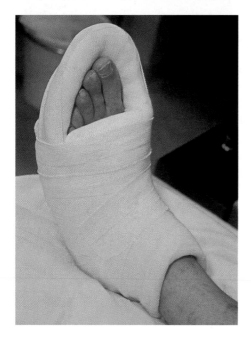

Figure 4.34
Pressure relief

A number of ways and devices have been used to relieve pressure and protect the foot in diabetes and other conditions (i.e. contact casting, Scotch cast boot, etc.). Shown in this photograph is the Blackburn boot, commonly used in the diabetes unit at the Blackburn Royal Infirmary. There are many steps to this procedure. Although these are time-consuming, it appears that this type of device is highly effective. Here one sees the final non-removable boot. One can also make the boot removable, which is a major advantage for some patients.

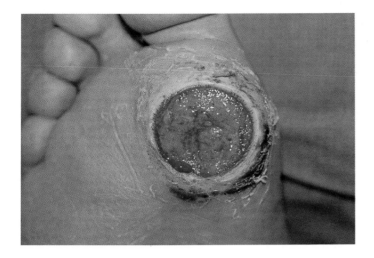

Figure 4.35a
Treating a non-healing diabetic ulcer

This man in his early 30's has severe neuropathy from diabetes, and his work does not allow him to adequately off-load. As a result, this neuropathic ulcer had not healed for 9 months. It is surrounded by a callus, which has a green color in some areas, suggesting hemorrhage and possible colonization with Pseudomonas bacteria. The obvious danger here is that the ulcer will become deeper and infected, which may require hospitalization, extensive surgery, or even amputation should osteomyelitis develop. The callus around this wound has to be removed in its entirety and the wound needs to be saucerized. This was done on a weekly basis and he was told to off-load as much as possible. Contact casting or Scotch cast boot would be a useful approach here, but was not practical for him.

Figure 4.35b
Treating a non-healing diabetic ulcer/Follow-up

He came to the office weekly, and we would remove the callus and reinforce the need for off-loading. The wound would be dressed with saline-soaked gauze. This photograph, taken several weeks later, shows that the ulcer is smaller, less deep, and has better granulation tissue. The formation of new callus suggests that he was unable to off-load adequately. There are some who believe, however, that callus keeps forming for several days or weeks, even after the patient is completely off-loaded.

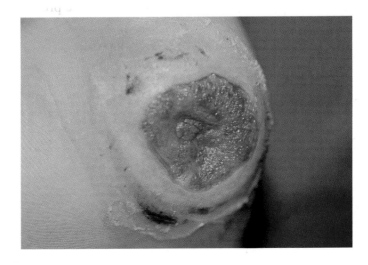

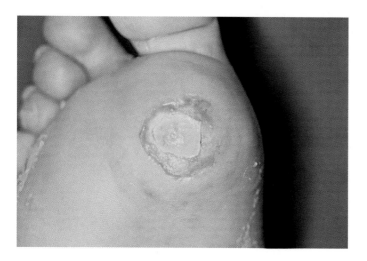

Figure 4.35c
Treating a non-healing diabetic ulcer/Use of bioengineered skin

The ulcer was improving but was slow in healing. We decided to use a bioengineered skin product (Graftskin) which consists of a bilayered construct of living keratinocytes and fibroblasts. Here one can see the bioengineered skin in place over the wound. In this case, the graft was trimmed to fit the wound, but in other cases we overlap the wound's edges; it has been hypothesized that the overlap can actually stimulate the cells at the periphery of the wound and accelerates healing. A few small cuts have been made in the bioengineered skin product before it was applied to the wound. These cuts allow the escape of wound fluid, which would otherwise accumulate under the graft and separate it from the wound bed.

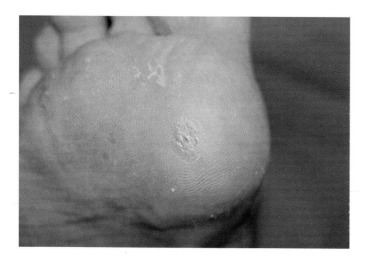

Figure 4.35d
Treating a non-healing diabetic ulcer/Healed wound

This photograph was taken about two months later. There has been complete healing of the wound and, so far, no recurrence. He is now wearing custom-fitted shoes. He must be seen periodically to inspect this healed area and other parts of his feet and, most importantly, to reinforce the need to off-load.

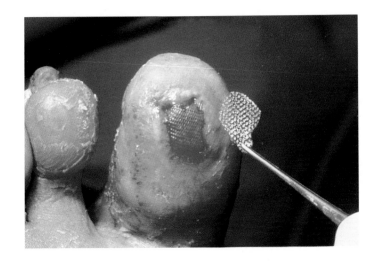

Figure 4.36
Other types of bioengineered skin

The field of bioengineered skin is emerging as a major force which will revolutionize the care of chronic wounds. In the previous examples, we have shown the use and effect of a bilayered living skin construct. In this photograph, the pressure ulcer on the big toe is being treated with a dermal skin substitute (Dermagraft®) consisting of human neonatal keratinocytes living in an absorbable matrix material. Besides the ones shown, there are already and we are likely to see other types of bioengineered skin constructs in the next few years. Some of these agents will be modifications of existing ones, i.e., adding endothelial cells, reengineering with certain growth factors or matrix gene constructs that are constitutively expressed or whose expression can be regulated by the wound environment.

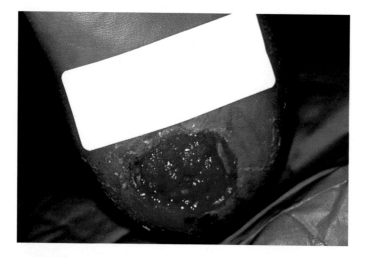

Figure 4.37a
Diabetic ulcers and dermal skin substitutes

This wound in a diabetic patient shows excellent granulation tissue and should heal with appropriate off-loading measures. Bioengineered skin products (in this case the dermal substitute shown in the previous photograph) can be used to accelerate the healing process.

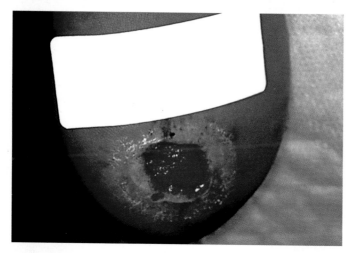

Figure 4.37b
Diabetic ulcers and dermal skin substitutes/Healing

This photograph was taken after 5 weeks of therapy. The ulcer has healed substantially and there is an 'edge' effect.

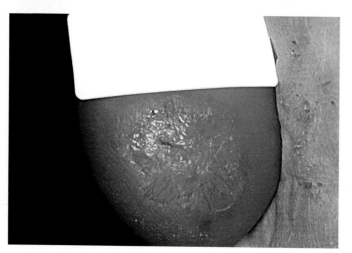

Figure 4.37c
Diabetic ulcers and dermal skin substitutes/Healed ulcer

After 10 weeks of therapy there has been complete healing of the ulceration. It is important to note that off-loading measures will need to be continued for the rest of this patient's life, or else he is likely to re-ulcerate.

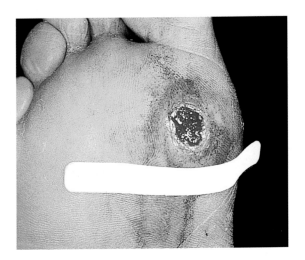

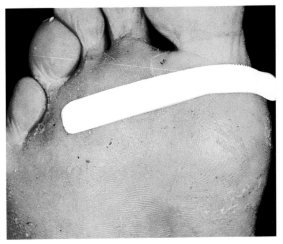

Figure 4.38a
**Platelet-derived growth factor
(PDGF)**

The topical application of this growth factor
0.01% gel preparation (becaplermin or
Regranex®) has been shown to enhance the
healing of diabetic neuropathic ulcers. It is
important that the wound be properly debrided
before starting treatment with PDGF.
Interestingly, there seems to be a synergistic
effect between proper surgical debridement and
use of PDGF. The neuropathic ulcer shown in
this photograph has just been debrided and the
surrounding callus removed. It has been stated
that this thorough debridement creates an
"acute wound" which is more responsive to
growth factor treatment.

Figure 4.38b
**Platelet-derived growth factor (PDGF)/After
treatment**

Complete healing of the ulceration has
occurred with becaplermin treatment. Please
note that there is little if any scarring and no
contraction. The use of growth factors has
proven safe, and adds to the number of
advanced therapeutic modalities now
available for diabetic ulcers.

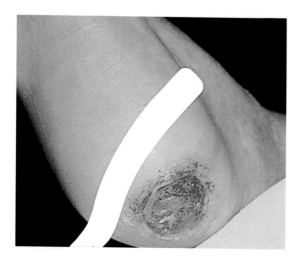

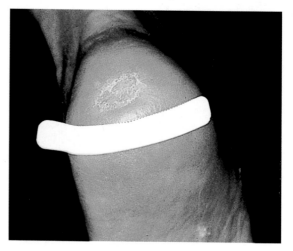

Figure 4.39a
Diabetic neuropathic ulcer in heel area

Heel ulcers in diabetic patients are often
problematic. Although in this case the ulcer
was mostly secondary to the neuropathy and
pressure, a vascular deficit often complicates
these ulcers. After debridement and wound
preparation, treatment was instituted with
topical PDGF, which is applied once daily.
The wound was irrigated with normal saline,
and a cotton applicator was used to apply
topical becaplermin gel as a thin continuous
layer. This is generally followed by a dressing
consisting of saline-moistened gauze which is
only in contact with the wound area. The
dressing is changed after 12 hours, but re-
application of the PDGF gel is only done
daily.

Figure 4.39b
**Diabetic neuropathic ulcer in heel
area/Complete closure**

After about 10 weeks of therapy there has
been complete healing of the ulceration. As
with any therapeutic modality, good wound
care (with periodic debridement if necessary)
and off-loading measures are critical to
obtaining good results.

5 Vascular ulcers

Introduction

Many ulcers occur on the extremities, and most of them are due to vascular problems. Therefore, not surprisingly, this section of our atlas is more extensive than the others. Included in this section are arterial, venous and lymphatic ulcers. We also discuss ulcers which are due to obstruction of small blood vessels with fibrin thrombi (i.e. cryofibrinogenemia and antiphospholipid syndrome).

Venous insufficiency is the most common etiology for ulcers of the lower extremity. The fundamental abnormality is venous hypertension, which refers to failure of the venous pressure to decrease in response to calf muscle pump action (e.g. during walking). Failure of the calf muscle pump could be due to a problem either with veins, such as retrograde bloodflow, or the calf muscles themselves, as in neurologic illness. We still do not fully understand how venous hypertension causes leg ulceration, but several hypotheses have been proposed. An early observation was that dermal capillaries in the fibrotic skin affected by venous disease (lipodermatosclerosis) were surrounded by fibrin cuffs. This led to the notion that venous hypertension causes leakage of fibrinogen, which then polymerizes to fibrin. It has been thought that the fibrin cuffs might reduce the proper exchange of oxygen and other nutrients between the dermis and blood. It remains unclear whether this "fibrin barrier" is truly operational in venous disease; it seems that the cuffs are incomplete around the dermal vessels. However, one could envision that, under conditions of poor microcirculation, fibrin could indeed act as a barrier. Most importantly, this hypothesis and subsequent studies showing defective tissue and systemic fibrinolysis in patients with venous disease has revived the idea of using fibrinolytic agents to treat venous ulcers.

Another interesting hypothesis for venous ulceration suggests that endothelial cells are damaged by venous hypertension, which then leads to adherence of circulating mononuclear cells, release of mediators, and further vascular permeability and tissue damage. Tumor necrosis factor-α (TNF-α) is probably one of these mediators. This hypothesis is also associated with clear therapeutic implications. For example, venous ulcers have been shown to heal faster with high systemic doses of pentoxifylline, which can inhibit the action of TNF-α. A third prominent hypothesis for venous ulcers proposes that macromolecular leakage (fibrinogen, albumin, α_2-macroglobulin) leads to trapping of growth factors within the wound. The idea here is that, although they are present in the wound, growth factors are no longer available for proper wound repair. Interestingly, α_2-macroglobulin is an established scavenger for growth factors and does leak into the dermis.

Within this section are examples of ulcers which cause considerable diagnostic difficulties, and which are characterized by obstruction of dermal capillaries with thrombi or other material (e.g. cholesterol emboli). Clinically, these ulcers present with areas of "microlivedo", purple discoloration of the foot and skin around the wound, and areas of dark necrotic tissue in the wound itself or at the edges. One of us (VF) has labeled ulcers having this clinical/histologic picture as "microthrombotic ulcers." Those that are due to cryofibrinogenemia may respond dramatically to the anabolic steroid stanozolol, in terms of both pain and ulcer healing. We present several examples of these conditions.

Stanozolol also seems to help the pain and other symptoms and signs of inflammation associated with acute (or early) lipodermatosclerosis. These patients often present with a picture resembling cellulitis but which is unresponsive to systemic antibiotics. We believe that this clinical condition is the acute counterpart of chronic lipodermatosclerosis. Patients with acute lipodermatosclerosis have evidence of venous insufficiency and will generally develop the intense fibrosis associated with long-standing venous disease. Ulcers often develop within the lipodermatosclerotic tissue.

In this section, we have also tried to dispel some of what we regard as clinical myths regarding venous and other types of ulcers. For example, venous ulcers are not invariably associated with hyperpigmentation in the surrounding skin, and the absence of this finding should not exclude a venous etiology for the ulcer. Pain is very commonly associated with venous ulcers, contrary to what students and doctors are generally taught. The verrucous changes associated with lymphedema can develop rather rapidly, within a few months after lymphatic obstruction. What looks like great granulation tissue in chronic vascular ulcers is not always desirable; it may represent infection or some other process (e.g. basal cell carcinoma). Split-thickness skin grafts are often used in the treatment of vascular ulcers. However, it is not fully appreciated how painful the donor sites can be; patients are very reluctant to undergo additional grafting procedures.

Other sections describe wound dressings in more detail. Here we give several examples of how compression bandages are applied. There has been considerable progress in the development of better and more effective compression bandages. Compression remains the established treatment for venous ulcers, but there is considerable controversy regarding what constitutes the ideal bandage. Some experts favor elastic compression, often multilayered, while others believe that rigid or semi-rigid (non-elastic) bandages are optimal. The majority of venous ulcers heal with compression therapy alone, and there is evidence that occlusive dressings may add to the beneficial effects of compression. There is increasing interest in methods or measurements which may allow us to predict which ulcers will go on to heal with these traditional and conservative methods. Recent work points to evidence of healing within the first 3–4 weeks as a very useful marker for complete healing several months later. This type of work is very important from a number of aspects. If confirmed, measurements of healing rates in the first few weeks could be used as a guide for the use of different treatment modalities, e.g. grafting. Also, it is possible that pilot clinical trials in the treatment of some chronic wounds could make use of healing rates within the first few weeks as surrogate markers to guide further drug development.

Bioengineered skin products will probably redefine the way in which we treat chronic wounds, including vascular ulcers. As with all new technologies, work is still required to identify how best to create and use such therapy. Here we give some examples of what might be expected with the use of bilayered skin constructs composed of living keratinocytes and fibroblasts. This type of treatment is very attractive because it allows clinicians to use living cells to modify the wound microenvironment. Increasing evidence points to abnormalities in the phenotype of cells within chronic wounds (e.g. increased senescence, unresponsiveness to some growth factors). Bioengineered skin products may work, at least in part, by providing new young cells which are "smart" and capable of adapting to the needs of the wound.

Clinical points

- The ankle/brachial index (ABI) is not reliable in patients with non-compressible arteries, as in diabetes.
- Biopsies are a safe and often necessary way to evaluate chronic wounds. Biopsy sites at the edges of the wound heal readily and often to the original margin.
- The presence of exposed tendons or a black eschar within a wound basically rules out a venous etiology.
- Microlivedo refers to a pattern of small linear streaks, often purple and not fully reticulated in configuration. It is associated with the formation of dermal thrombi, such as in cryofibrinogenemia and the antiphospholipid syndrome. We have labeled these conditions "micro-thrombotic ulcers".
- Venous insufficiency is the most common etiology for ulcers of the lower extremity.
- Acute lipodermatosclerosis is red and painful and resembles cellulitis. Occasionally, it is also mistaken for localized scleroderma (morphea). It responds dramatically to treatment with the anabolic steroid stanozolol.
- Compression bandages remain the established treatment for venous ulcers and should be part of any therapeutic program.
- When taking a biopsy from fibrotic skin, as in lipodermatosclerosis, a long and thin

excision closed primarily gives the best chance of healing. A punch biopsy can create an ulcer.
- Pericapillary fibrin deposition is a hallmark of lipodermatosclerosis and can be easily demonstrated by direct immunofluorescence.
- Arterial insufficiency should be suspected when ulcers are punched out or necrotic in appearance.
- Livedo reticularis is seen in 90% of patients with cholesterol embolization.
- Widespread cutaneous necrosis can be seen in a number of disease processes: connective tissue disease, vasculitis, disseminated intravascular coagulation (DIC).
- Venous ulcers do exist without the "typical" hyperpigmentation and lipodermatosclerosis surrounding the ulcer.
- Localized supplemental pressure is directly applied to ulcers that are in concave locations on the leg and where compression bandages are often not able to achieve optimal treatment.
- Multilayered bandages are preferred in patients whose legs have a "bowling pin" appearance. The non-compressive components can be used to "fill in" certain areas on the leg and thus allow the compression bandages to work better.
- When venous ulcers are in the "healing mode", the wound edges become flat and the epithelium begins to migrate towards the center.
- Dermatitis is a major therapeutic problem in patients with venous insufficiency. It remains unclear whether dermatitis is a true manifestation of venous disease or a complication of sensitization to topically applied agents.
- Lymphedema complicates many cases of venous disease. Chronic use of systemic

- antibiotics may sometimes be required to control the associated recurrent cellulitis.
- Sickle cell ulcers are probably due to both venous insufficiency and an arteriolar component. They do not respond readily to treatment. A comprehensive program of blood transfusion, grafting, hyperbaric oxygen and pentoxifylline may be necessary.
- Autologous grafting is an acceptable way to treat difficult-to-heal venous ulcers. Graft take is usually good, but it is important to maintain adequate compression for the grafts to spread and remain in the wound.
- Bioengineered skin is revolutionizing the way in which we treat difficult-to-heal venous ulcers. Actual initial take of the bioengineered skin is occasionally seen, but the main mode of action appears to be stimulation of healing.
- The "edge effect" refers to stimulation of the ulcer edge to start migrating and resurface the wound. Bioengineered skin often leads to an edge effect.

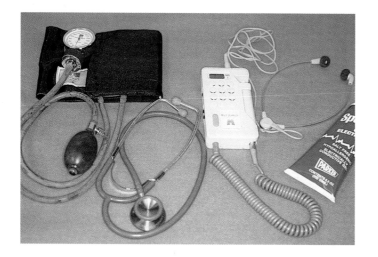

Figure 5.1a
Arterial Doppler testing

One can get quite sophisticated in testing patients for arterial disease and other vascular problems. Essential components, however, can be quite simple and relatively inexpensive. A blood pressure cuff, an arterial Doppler ultrasound and lubricating gel are basic requirements. Testing is done with the patient supine.

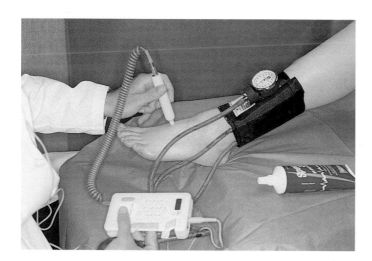

Figure 5.1b
Arterial Doppler testing/ABI

A blood pressure cuff is wrapped around the lower leg and the Doppler probe is placed over the dorsalis pedis artery. When the ultrasound signal is detected, the pressure cuff is inflated above the known systolic pressure to obliterate the Doppler sound. The cuff is then released slowly, and the level at which one can hear the Doppler sound is recorded. The same measurement is done with the brachial artery. The ankle to brachial index (ABI) is the ratio of the pressures obtained at the brachial artery and at the ankle, and is normally 1.1. Generally, a ratio above 0.7 or 0.8 indicates absence of significant arterial disease. At an ABI of around 0.5, one is probably dealing with a very serious situation that may require surgical reconstruction.

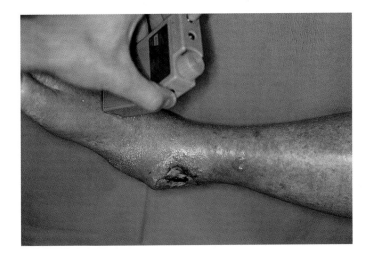

Figure 5.1c
Arterial Doppler testing/Arterial disease

In patients with significant arterial disease, even the Doppler device may be unable to locate a pulse. It should be noted that ABI measurements are not foolproof. Particularly in patients with diabetes, or others with non-compressible vessels, the ABI is an inadequate method for assessing arterial insufficiency. In such cases, color duplex scanning and pulse volume measurements may be indicated. Generally, these tests require referral to a vascular laboratory.

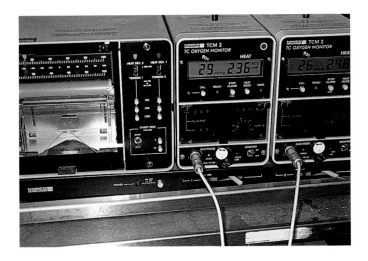

Figure 5.2a
Transcutaneous oxygen measurements ($TcPO_2$)

Devices such as this can measure the amount of oxygen diffusing through the skin. The $TcPO_2$ levels can be very valuable in assessing perfusion. In patients with diabetes and in need of amputation, these measurements have been used to decide on the level of amputation.

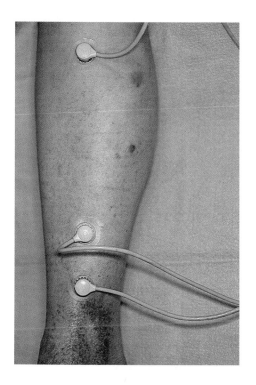

Figure 5.2b
Transcutaneous oxygen measurements (TcPO$_2$)

Measurements are made with sensors attached to electrodes, which connect with the type of device just shown. The skin sensor temperature is raised to around 42°C. At this temperature, the dermal vessels are maximally dilated. Multiple measurements can be made at one time. Usually, a control site, such as the infraclavicular area, is chosen to compare readings.

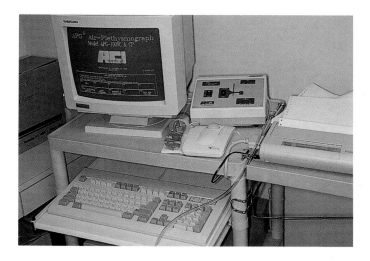

Figure 5.3a
Air plethysmography

This is an example of the type of equipment needed to perform this testing. Air plethysmography can be very useful in determining the extent of venous reflux and the function of the calf muscle pump. Properly done, serial measurements can be a reliable way to follow patients.

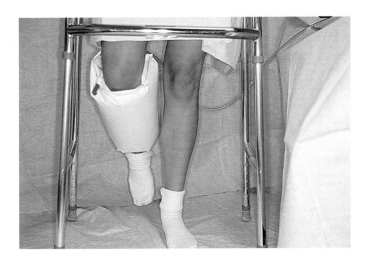

Figure 5.3b
Air plethysmography/Testing

For testing, patients go though a series of maneuvers: (1) supine and leg elevation to drain the venous system; (2) inflating and deflating the cuff after a series of foot dorsiflexions; (3) and the use of tourniquets to distinguish between superficial and deep vein components. What are available at the end are actual measurements of venous refilling time, volume ejection and other calculated variables. The data can be easily printed or stored in the computer.

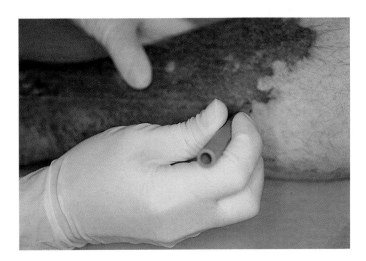

Figure 5.4a
Punch biopsies

These are done very commonly to study the ulcer itself or associated skin findings. Here a biopsy was done because the hyperpigmentation in this patient with venous ulcers was so very extensive and we wanted to exclude Kaposi's sarcoma.

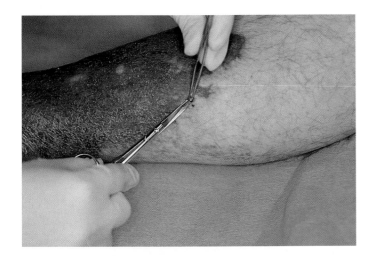

Figure 5.4b
Punch biopsies/Removal of skin

The small 3–4-mm cylindrical
piece of skin is removed with
forceps and scissors.

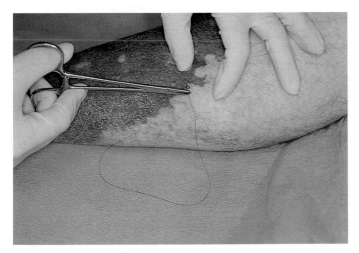

Figure 5.4c
Punch biopsies/Suturing

In general, we do not suture
biopsy sites from actual ulcers. In
this case, however, it is a good
idea to approximate the edges to
allow faster and more reliable
closure.

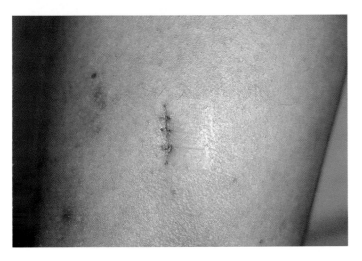

Figure 5.5
Excisional biopsy

In this case, an excisional biopsy
was done to obtain a specimen from
an area of lipodermatosclerosis
(LDS). Such biopsies from fibrotic
skin need to be very thin and long,
so as to allow easy closure without
much tension. If this is not done,
one often runs the risk of creating
an ulcer. As in this case, we supple-
ment the sutures with adhesive strips
and delay the removal of the sutures
by a few days.

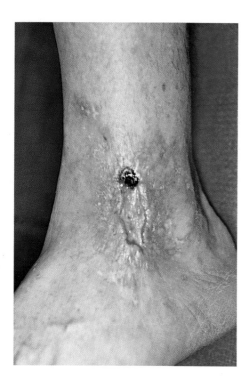

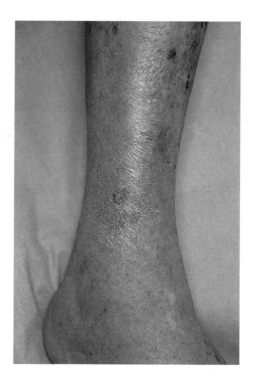

Figure 5.6
Ulcer biopsy

This ulcer was thought to be venous in etiology. However, the presence of subtle areas of microlivedo around the ulcer also suggested the possibility of cryofibrinogenemia. A biopsy was done to exclude dermal fibrin thrombi. This photograph was taken a week after the biopsy. It should be noted that biopsies of venous ulcers generally heal up to the original edge. Also, it is sometimes necessary to extend the biopsy a centimeter or more beyond the margins when one suspects the presence of malignancy.

Figure 5.7a
Testing closure with hydrogen peroxide

It has been reported that when hydrogen peroxide is applied to a wound, there will be a bubbling effect because of the serum present on the surface. Presumably this could be used to assess wound closure. The ulcer shown here is obviously not healed yet. We decided to apply a small drop of hydrogen peroxide to its base. Use of this test is not universally accepted.

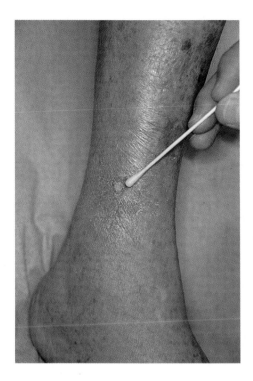

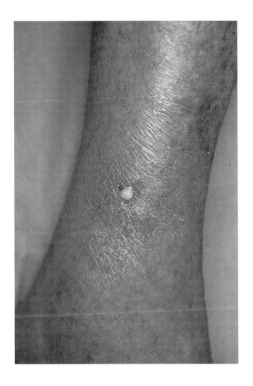

Figure 5.7b
Testing closure with hydrogen peroxide/Application

Here a cotton applicator is used to apply a small drop of hydrogen peroxide to the wound.

Figure 5.7c
Testing closure with hydrogen peroxide/Bubbling

As predicted, bubbling occurred within a few seconds. However, we have found that this reported way to assess complete wound closure is not foolproof. For example, bubbling occurs when the hydrogen peroxide is applied to an area containing residual scab or crust over a healed wound. Presumably, serum components are still present in the scab to allow this reaction to occur.

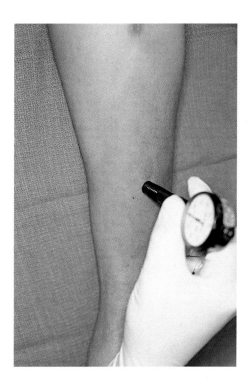

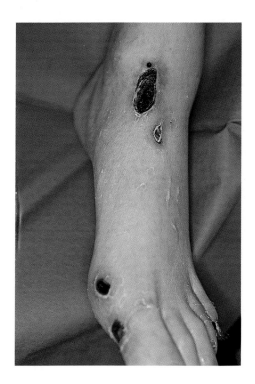

Figure 5.8
Use of durometer for testing skin hardness

This device has been traditionally used by engineers to measure the hardness of metals and plastics. We have adapted it for use in measuring skin hardness in various situations, including lipodermatosclerosis (as in this photograph). The test is easy and reproducible, but will give falsely elevated readings when the probe is applied directly over thin skin areas of the body; the hardness of the underlying bone is then detected. It is important to apply the device directly perpendicular to the skin and use gravity to hold it in place.

Figure 5.9
Arterial ulcers

In this 68-year-old man, these necrotic and punched-out ulcers appeared within a few weeks. He was found to have severe arterial insufficiency by angiography. The necrosis is a valuable clue. For example, venous ulcers would never have this type of black eschar. Embolization, i.e. chosterol emboli, could give a similar clinical picture but is generally associated with a livedo reticularis or micro-livedo pattern.

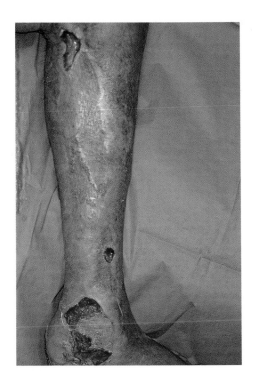

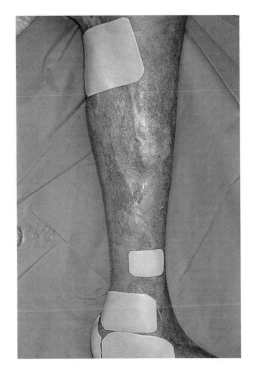

Figure 5.10a
Ulcers after arterial surgical reconstruction

This 52-year-old man with severe
claudication and arterial insufficiency was
surgically treated with a bypass procedure.
Shortly thereafter, he developed numerous
ulcerations, in spite of adequate pulses. Some
of these ulcers were near grafted sites.

Figure 5.10b
Ulcers after arterial surgical reconstruction

His bloodflow was adequate and good
wound care should enable these ulcers to
heal. He was treated with hydrocolloid
dressings. A few months later, he was
completely healed. We have seen patients
develop ulcers after surgical reconstruction,
particularly within the surgical excisions.
Often, conservative therapy or even small
grafts can help the situation.

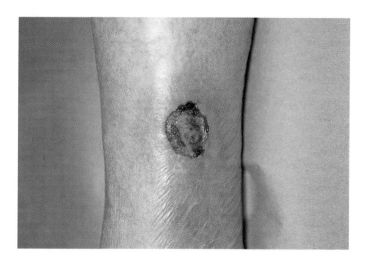

Figure 5.11
Ulcer with necrotic edges

Arterial insufficiency should be considered whenever there is an element of severe necrosis and eschar. In this case, however, the diagnosis was pyoderma gangrenosum, which is often associated with systemic conditions, such as inflammatory bowel disease and rheumatoid arthritis.

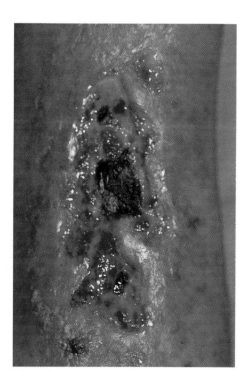

Figure 5.12
Eschar in ulcer bed

Again, the presence of an eschar argues against venous disease. There is also no hyperpigmentation, which is a hallmark of venous disease. The patient is an 82-year-old woman with widespread atherosclerosis and inoperable peripheral vascular disease. This tibial ulcer was very painful. The pain did not respond to pentoxifylline and to occlusive dressings. She required narcotic analgesics to control the pain. We have found the topical use of anesthetics under occlusion, such as EMLA, to be helpful. This case also illustrates the fact that, while often effective, occlusive dressings do not always relieve pain. Another therapeutic approach to improve pain here would be the use of grafts or bioengineered skin.

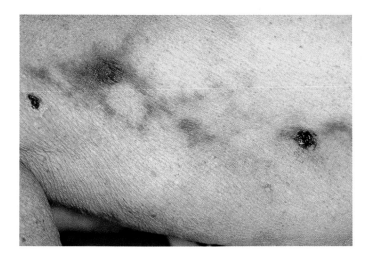

Figure 5.13
Calciphylaxis

This 62-year-old woman presented with painful livedo-like lesions in the setting of renal failure. The livedo, the necrotic areas and the clinical setting are highly suggestive of calciphylaxis. A biopsy showed calcium deposition in and around the vessel walls. These patients have a high mortality, and calciphylaxis often occurs as an end-stage event. Calcium channel blockers have been advocated as a treatment.

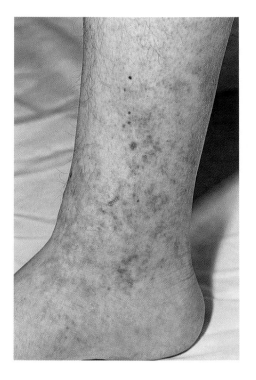

Figure 5.14
Cholesterol embolization

The clinical hallmark of cholesterol embolization is livedo reticularis, which is present in up to 90% of patients. Ulcerations of toes and legs are not uncommon. The condition occurs as a result of dislodging of atherosclerotic material from atheromas, either spontaneously, or after angiography, or even after treatment with warfarin. The less than 100-μm emboli obstruct the microcirculation and give a clinical picture of livedo reticularis and ulcers, and systemic disease (especially kidney and brain). Interestingly, the blood pressure is usually normal in these cases, and peripheral pulses are palpable. Biopsies from skin can reveal the typical cholesterol clefts in subcutaneous vessels, but serial sectioning of biopsy specimens may be necessary.

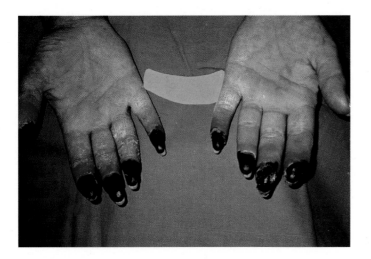

Figure 5.15
Massive necrosis of fingertips

This type of fulminant presentation is often associated with connective tissue diseases, such as rheumatoid arthritis. It generally represents a vasculitis, but coagulopathies may coexist or even be the primary cause. The patient improved considerably with systemic immunosuppressive therapy and wound debridement. She did not lose function of her hands or fingers.

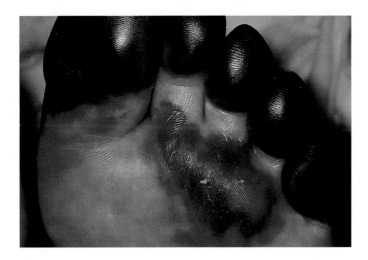

Figure 5.16a
Disseminated intravascular coagulation (DIC)

DIC is a serious complication of sepsis (i.e. meningococcemia), generalized infections (i.e. varicella), or widespread malignancy. The cutaneous necrosis can be so extensive as to require multiple amputations. Toes, fingers or entire extremities may become gangrenous. In this 42-year-old man with falciparum malaria, hemorrhagic blisters developed on toes, fingers, and some truncal areas.

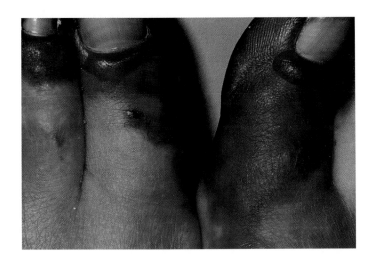

Figure 5.16b
Disseminated intravascular coagulation (DIC)/Hemorrhagic blisters

This process can evolve rather quickly, sometimes in a matter of hours. It often becomes necessary to debride necrotic areas extensively.

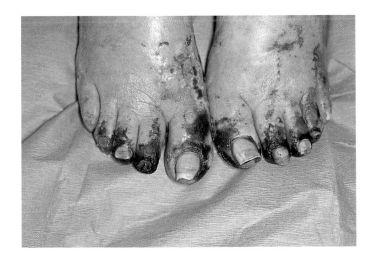

Figure 5.17a
Widespread necrosis in Hansen's disease (leprosy)

The patient developed necrosis of his fingertips and toes, together with extensive necrosis of truncal areas. He was in his 40s and had leprosy. This clinical picture represents Lucio's phenomenon, a serious reaction associated with ulceration, especially on the legs. Patients with lepromatous leprosy may develop erythema nodosum leprosum, while those with diffuse lepromatosis, as in this case, may develop Lucio's phenomenon.

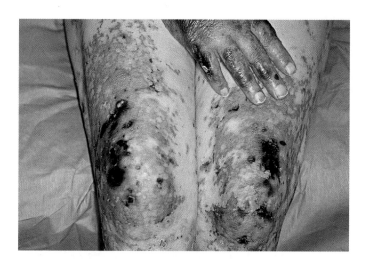

Figure 5.17b
Widespread necrosis (leprosy)/Livedo and ulcerations

Extensive necrosis and ulcerations around the knees. These lesions were very painful.

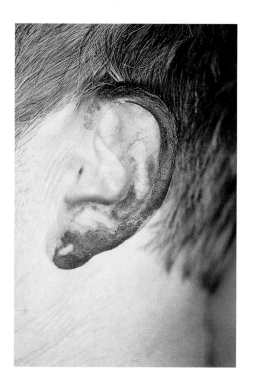

Figure 5.17c
Widespread necrosis (leprosy)/Generalized involvement

Distal areas are particularly prone to this complication of leprosy. Here one sees necrosis of the ear. The patient was treated with dapsone, rifampin, and clofazamine, and made a remarkable recovery.

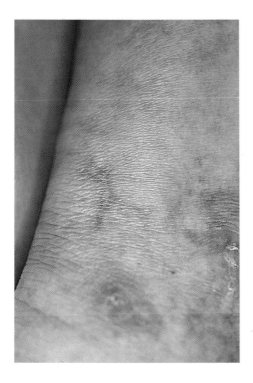

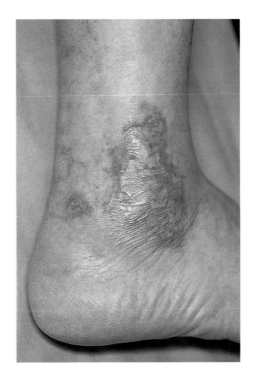

Figure 5.18a
Livedo pattern (microlivedo)

These are subtle findings. Instead of the intense livedo reticularis which, like a net, involves a large area of skin, one often sees faint linear streaks which are purple and do not form a complete "net". These lesions have been called "microlivedo" and are commonly observed on the lower leg and foot in cases of obstruction of small vessels.

Figure 5.18b
Livedo pattern (microlivedo)

The pattern of microlivedo is worth looking for when evaluating ulcers of the lower extremity. Microlivedo is not a specific clinical finding, and can be seen with cholesterol embolization, vasculitis, the antiphospholipid syndrome, cryofibrinogenemia, cryoglobulinemia and septic embolization. Biopsies and blood studies are necessary to look for these specific conditions. In this particular patient the ulcers were due to cryofibrinogenemia. His plasma showed cryofibrinogen and a biopsy of the large ulcer (which is now healed) showed the typical fibrin thrombi in small dermal vessels, without much inflammation. He was successfully treated with the anabolic steroid stanozolol.

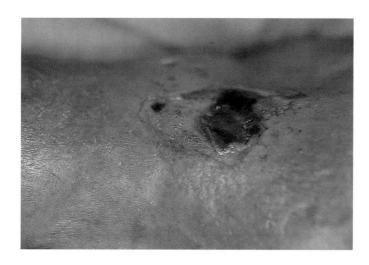

Figure 5.19
Ulcer due to microthrombi

The necrosis (eschar) and the lack of hyperpigmentation argue against a venous etiology. This patient too had dermal micro-thrombi but there was no associated laboratory abnormality (i.e. cryofibrinogen, anticardiolipin antibodies). In such cases, we have said that these patients have an idiopathic form of micro-thrombotic disease, which we call livedoid vasculitis. He improved with surgical debridement, wound care with hydrocolloids, and stanozolol. There have been reports of successfully using systemic tissue plasminogen activator (tPA) in such cases.

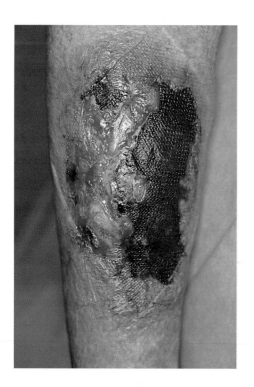

Figure 5.20
A dramatic case of cryofibrinogenemia

Again, the extensive necrosis is a clue and the pain is rather typical in that it is excruciating and is peculiarly relieved by gently rubbing the surrounding skin. He was an elderly man with many other medical problems, including congestive heart failure. He was admitted to the hospital and treated with stanozolol. One must be very cautious when giving stanozolol to patients with congestive heart failure or hypertension.

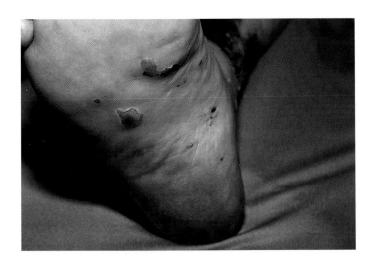

Figure 5.21
Vasculitis resembling septic emboli

This 38-year-old man had fevers, arthralgia, and cutaneous lesions which were initially thought to represent septic emboli. However, there was no evidence of endocarditis, and the biopsy showed leucocytoclastic vasculitis. The vasculitis may have been due to antibiotics he had taken for an unrelated problem.

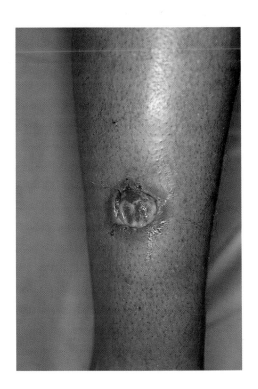

Figure 5.22
Vasculitis due to rheumatoid arthritis

The edges are purple and, in the setting of rheumatoid arthritis, the initial thought was that this may represent pyoderma gangrenosum. However, a biopsy showed vasculitis. The patient required treatment with systemic corticosteroids.

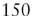

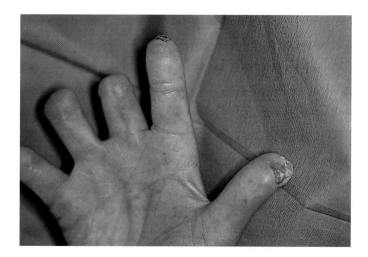

Figure 5.23a
Scleroderma ulcers

This 48-year-old man with the CREST variant of systemic sclerosis (scleroderma) has had numerous ulcerations which have resulted in autoamputation of several digits. The ulceration on his right thumb has been present for several months and is being treated with cadexomer iodine, which has helped the exudation and has led to considerable healing. On his palms, one can see the typical matted telengiectasia that are associated with the CREST syndrome. Patients such as this develop early vascular damage, such as intimal proliferation. Because of the obstructive nature of these vascular lesions, they do not respond well to vasodilators.

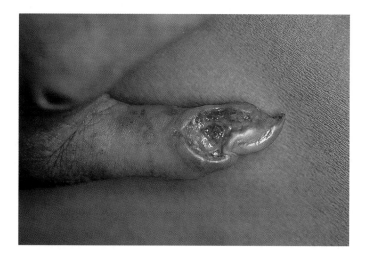

Figure 5.23b
Scleroderma ulcers/Partial healing

This other patient also has systemic sclerosis (scleroderma) and persistent digital ulcers. The thumb ulceration seen here was treated with a hydrogel, which was able to manage the exudate, stimulate granulation tissue, and relieve some of the pain. Her clinical course was complicated by frequent bouts of infection. It is often difficult to tell whether sudden worsening of these ulcers is due to infection or more ischemia. If antibiotics need to be used, they probably have to be administered for prolonged periods of time.

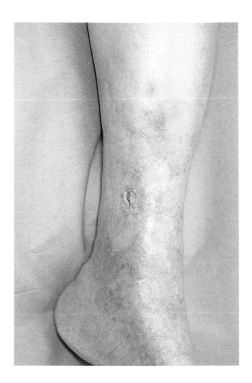

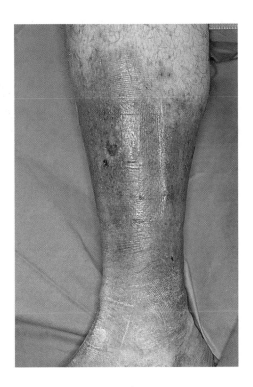

Figure 5.24
Acute (early) lipodermatosclerosis (LDS)

This 58-year-old woman had persistent pain in her leg for over a year. Some clinicians thought she might have localized scleroderma (morphea). Because of recurrent bouts of worsening pain associated with redness, she was hospitalized multiple times for treatment of presumed cellulitis. Actually, this clinical course is very familiar to us. These patients have acute (or early) LDS, which is associated with venous insufficiency. It represents a panniculitis and responds rather dramatically to treatment with the anabolic steroid stanozolol. In our experience, most of these patients cannot use graded stockings because of the pain. The ulcer in the middle of the fibrotic plaque was due to a punch biopsy. It is best to perform excisional biopsies in these patients and close them primarily.

Figure 5.25
Acute and painful lipodermatosclerosis (LDS)

This 55-year-old woman with associated cardiovascular disease has redness and warmth associated with LDS. Not surprisingly, many of these patients are thought to have cellulitis. She is being treated with compression bandages and has been able to tolerate this treatment. Because of her cardiovascular disease, we were afraid of using stanozolol, which can cause sodium retention and worsening of hypertension and congestive heart failure.

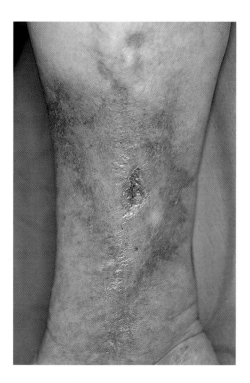

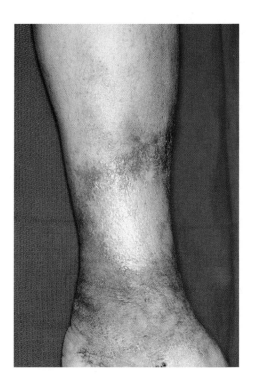

Figure 5.26
Chronic lipodermatosclerosis (LDS) with ulcer

This patient is in her 60s and has had venous insufficiency for many years. The fibrotic component involving most of the medial leg is generally painless and is not tender. It represents the chronic form of LDS. Ulcers develop within LDS and recur within LDS, and their failure to heal correlates with the severity of LDS. Trauma is often a precipitating event in causing the ulcers.

Figure 5.27
Chronic lipodermatosclerosis (LDS)

This patient has had multiple ulcerations which have healed with compression therapy. Note the prominent varicosities and areas of atrophie blanche. She remains on graded stockings, which will need to be used for the rest of her life. Chronic LDS often has this sharply demarcated border. A useful clinical finding is for the clinician to palpate the skin several centimeters above the superior edge of the hard plaque. A characteristic "cliff" with a sharp separation between the softer skin above and the hard skin below will be felt. This observation can also be made in the more acute presentations of LDS.

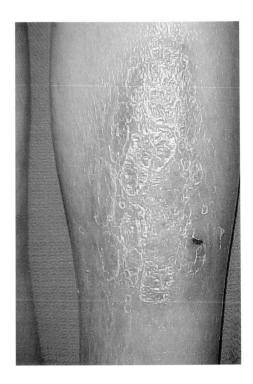

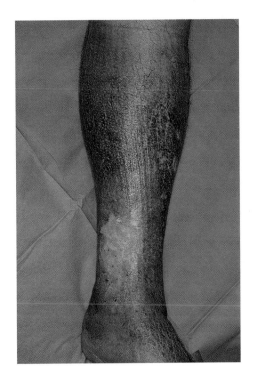

Figure 5.28
Lipodermatosclerosis and dermatitis

In colder climates, the clinical picture of venous disease can be somewhat different in that the involved skin is dry and scaly. This 82-year-old man had a very distinctive scaly plaque on his shin, which was not painful or tender. These plaques were present bilaterally, and we also thought of the possibility of pretibial myxedema. However, a biopsy showed no evidence of increased dermal deposition of hyaluronic acid and there were typical histologic findings of venous disease (i.e. increased tortuous vessels, hemosiderin deposition).

Figure 5.29
Healed ulcer and chronic lipodermatosclerosis (LDS)

The hypopigmented area on the medial aspect of the lower leg is an ulcer that has healed recently. Interestingly, it takes several months or even years for the pigment to return to the previously ulcerated site. The surrounding hyperpigmentation and the hardness of the skin are classic for chronic lipodermatosclerosis. There is usually little pain at this point, although some discomfort can be felt upon prolonged walking. This 64-year-old man needs to wear graded compression stockings for the rest of his life, so as to avoid recurrence of the ulcer.

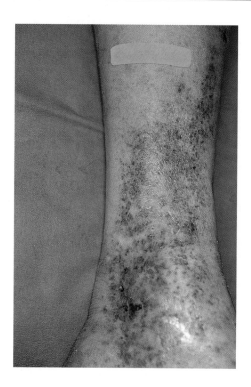

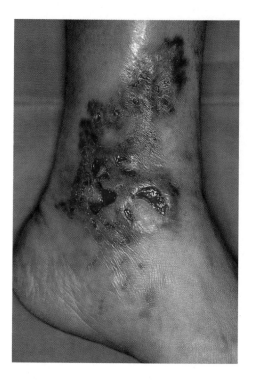

Figure 5.30
Lipodermatosclerosis and pain

The separation between acute and chronic
lipodermatosclerosis is somewhat artificial.
There are patients who have a more subacute
course, such as this person. She has areas of
induration (around the small ulcer) as well as
other features of venous disease; these
features have been present for years. She has
white atrophic lesions studded with
prominent small blood vessels (atrophie
blanche). It has been stated that patients with
venous insufficiency go through a clinical
course of either lipodermatosclerosis or
atrophie blanche. This may be true to a
certain extent, but in our experience some
patients have both conditions.

Figure 5.31a
**Unusual presentation of lipodermatosclerosis
(LDS) and ulcers**

This 34-year-old woman sustained an injury
at work and developed painful and highly
inflammatory lesions with ulcerations. The
history of trauma did not fit with the clinical
observations, and we thought she might have
a vasculitis or small vessel obstructive disease
from cryoproteins. However, her laboratory
studies were normal and several biopsies
from the inflamed and ulcerated areas were
most consistent with venous disease and
LDS.

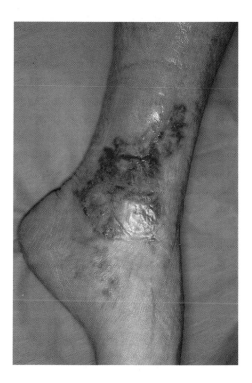

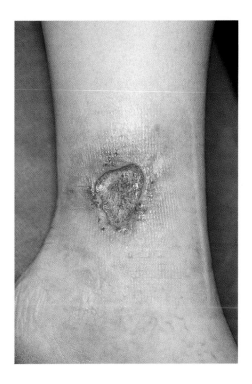

Figure 5.31b
Unusual presentation of lipodermatosclerosis (LDS and ulcers/After healing

Although initially treated with stanozolol, this patient did not respond to this therapy alone even at a higher dose of 8 mg/day. Her ulcers, however, did heal with foam dressings and compression therapy over a period of about 4 months. The stanozolol was tapered slowly over the next several months. The photograph shows that the ulcers have healed and that there is less inflammation. Stanozol, while helpful in several clinical situations, does not accelerate the healing of venous ulcers.

Figure 5.32a
Venous ulcer without hyperpigmentation

Many clinicians are used to the idea that most venous ulcers are surrounded by hyperpigmented skin and would doubt a venous etiology for an ulcer in the absence of such pigment. We think this is an oversimplification. There are patients with definite venous disease and ulceration in whom, for some reason, the hemosiderin deposition either does not occur or does not lead to eventual melanin production. This 34-year-old woman had a very serious deep vein thrombosis in this leg several years ago, which resulted in pulmonary embolism. The skin around the ulcer is hard, as in chronic lipodermatosclerosis (LDS).

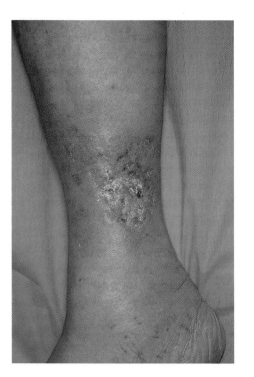

Figure 5.32b
Venous ulcer without hyperpigmentation/Not uncommon

In this other patient with proven venous insufficiency, there are increased varicosities and there is hardness of the medial aspect of the leg, as seen in lipodermatosclerosis (LDS). She too, however, lacks the "typical" hyperpigmentation surrounding the ulcer. Histologically, there were no other findings to suggest alternative diagnoses. Venous color duplex scanning showed venous insufficiency of both the superficial and deep system. She is healing on compression therapy alone.

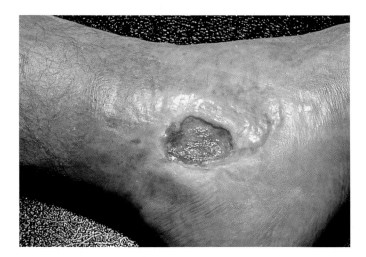

Figure 5.33
Typical venous ulcers

Most clinicians are used to this more classic presentation of a venous ulcer. In this 62-year-old man with proven venous insufficiency (by color duplex scanning) the skin is hyperpigmented and the ulcer has the typical irregular borders. This ulcer has been present for over 10 years. Note how the edges are steep, with a sharp cut-off between the edges and the ulcer bed. We say that these ulcers are not in a "healing mode". When the ulcer begins to heal, the edges become flattened and the epithelium begins to migrate.

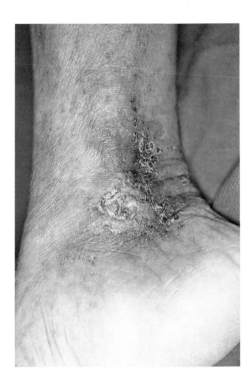

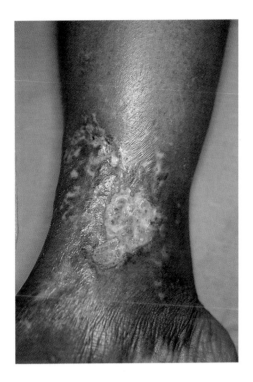

Figure 5.34
Another typical venous ulcer

The surrounding hyperpigmentation is what
one expects in venous ulcers. Although
rather small, this ulcer was very painful and
was not responding to treatment with
compression bandages. Ulcers such as this,
near or below the medial malleolus, are more
resistant to therapy with compression
bandages. It might very well be that
compression, as it is generally applied, does
not take into account the concave nature of
this location. Therefore, it is important to
use "fillers" such as extra dressings or wool
wraps to make this area more cylindrical
before applying compression.

Figure 5.35
**Venous insufficiency and systemic lupus
erythematosus (SLE)**

This patient began having leg ulcers at age
24, at about the time she was diagnosed as
having SLE. Now, almost 20 years later, she
continues to have recurrent ulcerations.
Clinically, some of the features (i.e. hyperpigmentation, irregular ulcers, hard skin) are
suggestive of venous ulcers. However, many
of the ulcers are small and punched-out and
resemble ulcerations due to vasculitis or the
antiphospholipid syndrome. She has venous
insufficiency (both superficial and deep vein)
and a biopsy of the ulcers showed changes
most consistent with venous disease (i.e.
tortuous blood vessels, hemosiderin
deposition). She had no cryoproteins or
anticardiolipin antibodies and improved with
compression bandages. This case illustrates
the fact that it is difficult sometimes to have
a definite diagnosis, and one may need to
rely on the response to treatment.

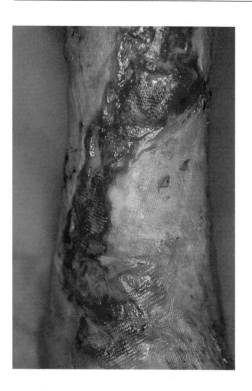

Figure 5.36
Unusual venous ulcer

Along the lines of atypical venous ulcers, this one too has unusual features. There is no hyperpigmentation but the ulcer is located in an area of intense lipodermatosclerosis (LDS). The shape of the ulcer is also unusual, because it is narrow and long. The undulating edges point to the possibility of a rheumatoid ulcer, but she did not have rheumatoid arthritis or other connective tissue diseases. She did not have plasma or serum cryoproteins (i.e. cryoglobulin, cryofibrinogen) and a biopsy did not show vasculitis. She improved dramatically with compression therapy. The edges here are seen to be in a "healing mode" in that they are flat and flush with the ulcer bed. Many of the translucent areas in the ulcer bed represent new epithelium.

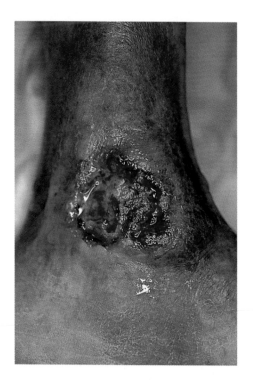

Figure 5.37
Ulcer with purple edges and venous insufficiency

This 59-year-old woman has venous insufficiency and lipodermatosclerosis (LDS) involving the lower leg. The ulcer is in the medial aspect of the leg. Taken together, these clinical findings suggest that the ulcer is venous in etiology. Although she eventually responded to hydrocolloid dressings and compression bandages, we could not be absolutely certain that this was a venous ulcer. The edges are purple, as in pyoderma gangrenosum, and the inferior border is necrotic, as we see in vasculitis, cryoproteinemias, or the antiphospholipid syndrome. However, laboratory testing could not confirm any of these possibilities, and the biopsy was more consistent with venous disease.

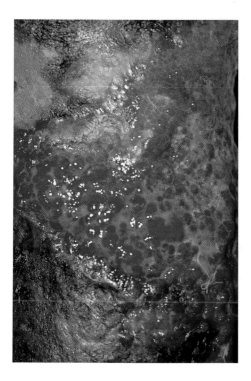

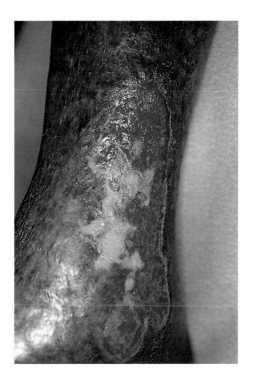

Figure 5.38
Venous ulcer and exuberant granulation tissue

There is overgrowth of granulation tissue which occurred after the use of an occlusive dressing. We do use occlusive dressings to create a moist wound environment and to promote granulation tissue, but we would regard this extent of granulation tissue as undesirable. Some believe that bacterial overgrowth may be responsible for exuberant granulation tissue. However, it should be noted that the superior edge is in a "healing mode", because it is flat and flush with the ulcer bed, while the lower edge shows absence of healing. This case also illustrates the fact that different areas of ulcers can be in different stages of healing. This patient was treated with a foam dressing and compression, which creates a less moist environment.

Figure 5.39
Venous ulcer in different stages of healing

There are several points for discussion here. First, the upper portion and mid-portion of the ulcer are healing well and the edge is flat (in a "healing mode"). In fact, the hypopigmented skin represents areas that have recently re-epithelialized. The inferior and more dependent part of the ulcer shows poor granulation tissue and a steeper edge (not in a "healing mode"). Although the tendency has been to dress wounds with one type of dressing, one can see here that the needs are different in these two areas of ulceration. One could use a protective foam dressing in the upper part and a hydrocolloid dressing to stimulate debridement and better granulation tissue in the lower part of the ulcer.

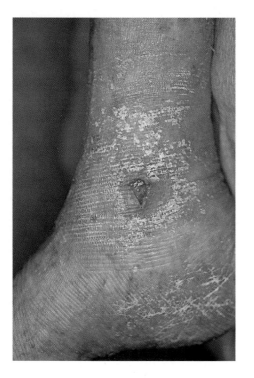

Figure 5. 40
Venous ulcer resistant to treatment with compression

Some ulcers, like this one, are small but do not heal readily with compression bandages. This 82-year-old woman has not responded to elastic or non-elastic compression. A common denominator for these small non-healing ulcers is that they are present near or below the malleolus. This site is difficult to wrap in a way that achieves proper compression. The concave areas need to be "filled" with other dressing material before compression is applied.

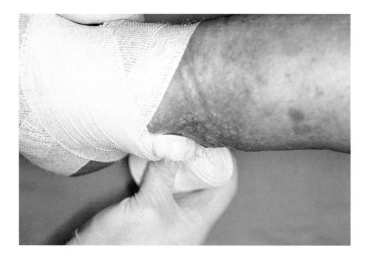

Figure 5.41
Venous ulcer and supplemental pressure

An easy way to circumvent the problem of applying proper compression to concave areas of the leg is to use extra gauze or foam dressings over the ulcer before compression is applied. We call this "localized supplemental pressure".

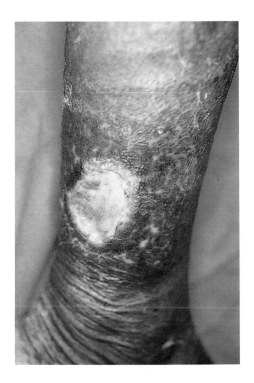

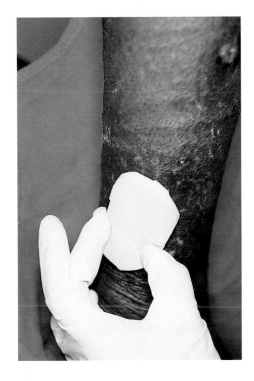

Figure 5.42a
Venous ulcer with foam supplemental pressure

We use localized supplemental pressure also when the ulcer is not healing, irrespective of its location. This 59-year-old woman has a venous ulcer that has not developed good granulation tissue and is not healing. Frequent surgical debridements have been required.

Figure 5.42b
Venous ulcer with foam supplemental pressure/Foam pressure

The foam dressing is cut to size and placed directly over the ulcer. This may help by creating greater pressures over the ulcer when the compression bandage is applied over it.

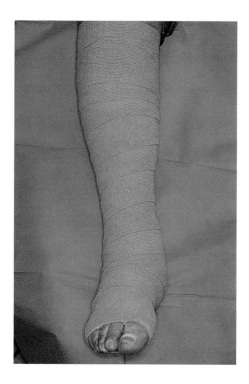

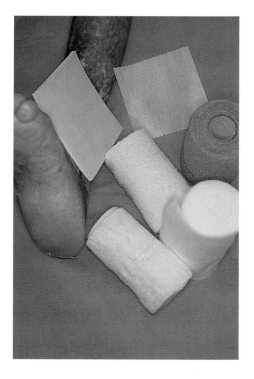

Figure 5.43
Venous ulcer and compression bandages

This photograph shows a self-adherent
elastic bandage in place from the toes to just
below the knee. Underneath it is a non-
elastic zinc-impregnated bandage (Unna
boot). This combination has become popular
in the USA, while many European countries
prefer multi-layered compression bandages.

Figure 5.44a
Multi-layered compression bandages

As mentioned above, these compression
systems are popular in Europe and
increasingly used in the USA. They are
composed of a primary dressing, the nature
of which is variable (i.e. a foam, a nylon
membrane), and three to four additional
bandages. High resting and working pressure
develop under these compression bandages.

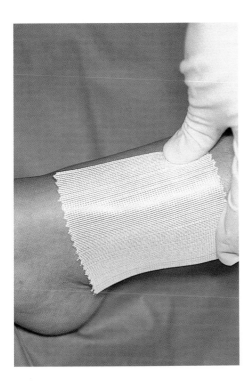

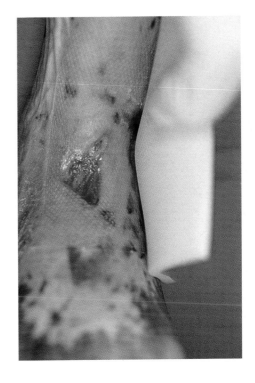

Figure 5.44b
Multi-layered compression bandages/Primary dressing

One possible primary dressing is shown here. It is non-adherent and non-absorbent. Some clinicians prefer to use a hydrocolloid as the primary dressing to keep a moist wound environment.

Figure 5.44c
Multi-layered compression bandages/Alternative primary dressing

If the ulcer is highly exudative, a foam dressing or a calcium alginate material could be used as the primary dressing.

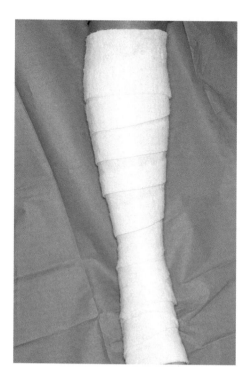

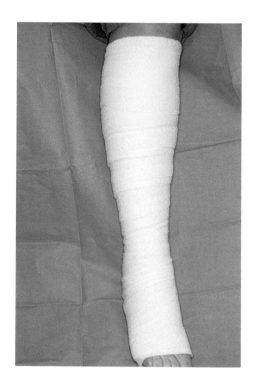

Figure 5.44d
Multi-layered compression bandages/First layer

This material, similar to those used under casts, is applied in a spiral fashion with a 50% overlap. It protects the leg, provides some padding, and can shape the leg in such a way that compression is applied more evenly. This is particularly important in legs that are very narrow at the ankle. In those cases, this material is used to "fill in" these areas and make the leg more cylindrical.

Figure 5.44e
Multi-layered compression bandages/Second layer

The second non-compressive layer is also applied in a spiral fashion with a 50% overlap. It is non-adherent and does not stretch very much. It holds the previous layer nicely in place and it keeps it smooth.

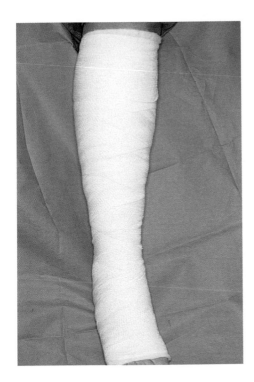

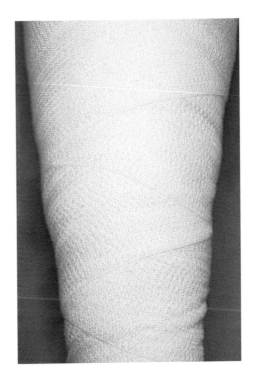

Figure 5.44f
Multi-layered compression bandages/Third layer

This compressive layer is applied in a figure of eight, which tends to prevent slippage.

Figure 5.44g
Multi-layered compression bandages/Third layer/Close-up

The figure of eight pattern is well seen here.

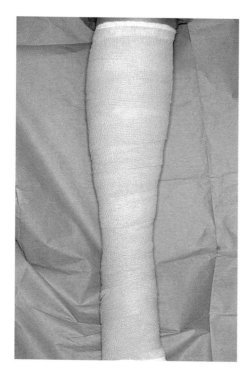

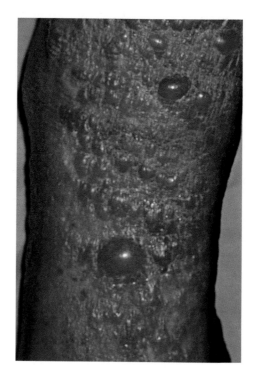

Figure 5.44h
Multi-layered compression bandages/Fourth layer

The fourth, like the third, is also a compression bandage but is applied in a spiral fashion with a 50% overlap. These systems are usually replaced once or twice a week depending on the needs of the patient and the amount of exudate.

Figure 5.45
Contact dermatitis and venous disease

This patient was being treated with an Unna boot and developed a bullous eruption thought to represent a contact dermatitis. This is not common, but would lead one to use elastic bandages instead in patients with known sensitivities to topical agents. It is important to realize that patients with venous disease have a high potential for contact sensitization.

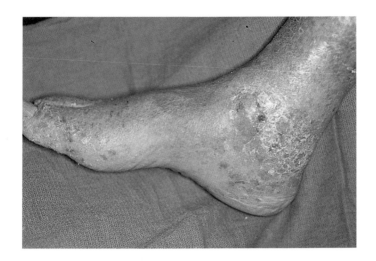

Figure 5.46
Dermatitis and swollen toes

Multi-layered bandages are a good way to deliver compression in patients with venous insufficiency and ulcers. Because of their high resting pressures, however, elastic bandages should be used cautiously in patients with known concomitant lymphatic disease. This 75-year-old man with a venous ulcer and lymphatic disease developed a substantial dermatitis and swollen toes after repeated application of high elastic compression. We have observed this problem in a few patients. In some cases, it has not been possible to apply any type of compression because of this complication. Pneumatic pumps are a useful alternative.

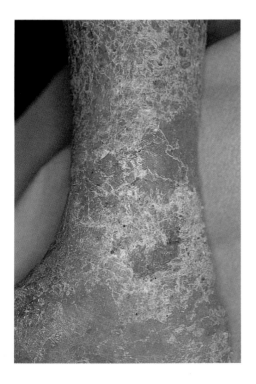

Figure 5.47
Contact dermatitis in venous disease

As mentioned earlier, patients with venous disease are particularly susceptible to contact dermatitis. Clinicians have always thought that "stasis" dermatitis is an intrinsic component of venous disease. However, we have recently come to the conclusion that "stasis" dermatitis may not be a real entity but the result of sensitization to topical agents. Once patients stop using the offending drug, it may take months before the dermatitis improves.

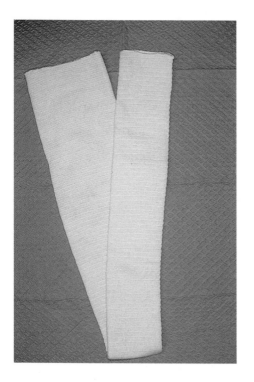

Figure 5.48
Shaped support bandages

When ulcers have healed and patients do not yet have elastic stockings, it is still necessary to provide compression so as to avoid ulcer recurrence. In some cases, we simply continue the compression bandages until stockings are obtained. In other cases, it may be possible to use the shaped support bandages shown here. These ready-to-wear graduated bandages can be very useful in the management of healed patients.

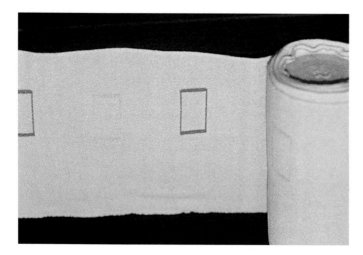

Figure 5.49a
Other compression bandages

There are a variety of compression devices on the market that are useful and effective in the treatment of venous ulcers. Some are very clever, like the one shown here. This elastic bandage has rectangles on its surface which, when stretched to the appropriate tension, become squares.

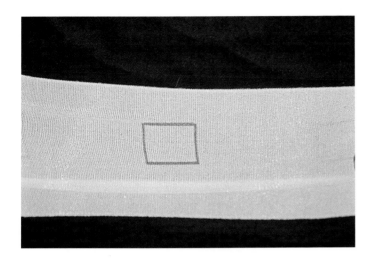

Figure 5.49b
**Other compression
bandages/Stretched**

The photograph shows how the
previous bandage looks after
stretching. This visualization of
the degree of tension promotes
more consistent and reliable
compression.

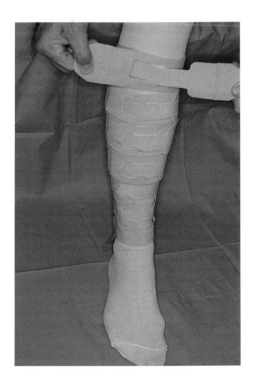

Figure 5.50
Alternative compression method

This device represents another way to achieve
compression, either during treatment of venous
ulcers, or if patients are unable to tolerate or apply
elastic stockings. These units shown in the
photograph are applied individually, from toes to
below the knee. There is a backstrip that is behind
the leg to which the individual units attach by means
of a velcro material. In this picture, only the ankle-
to-knee units have been applied so far. She will then
add the other components to complete the
application from the toes up.

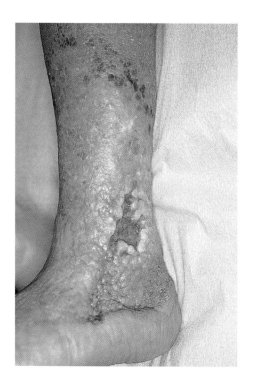

Figure 5.51a
Venous and lymphatic disease

This ulcer is probably of mixed venous and lymphatic etiology, not an uncommon combination. In fact, it has been reported that some degree of lymphatic obstruction is present in most patients with advanced venous insufficiency. The clinical features telling us that there is lymphatic disease are the presence of these verrucous changes and the fact that the leg is more cylindrical and does not have the "inverted bowling pin" appearance that is so common in venous disease.

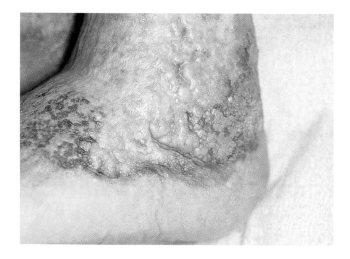

Figure 5.51b
Venous and lymphatic disease/Close-up

The skin is thrown into folds and there are fissures. Many clinicians often begin treating these patients with compression bandages, but this therapy can sometimes result in substantial edema of the toes. Compression pumps are often required to avoid this complication.

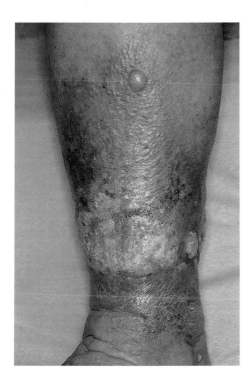

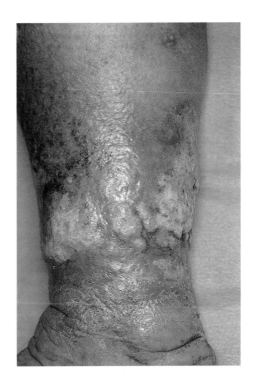

Figure 5.52a
Lymphedema and infection

Cellulitis and erysipelas are very common complications of lymphatic obstruction. As in this 62-year-old man, the cellulitis is often recurrent. In some cases, "chronic" cellulitis develops. The lymphatic system is probably so damaged that bacteria cannot be properly handled and cleared. Chronic systemic antibiotics have been used to prevent recurrences of the cellulitis. The photograph also shows a blister superiorly and a large anterior area of early breakdown. Leg elevation and systemic antibiotics are needed at this point.

Figure 5.52b
Lymphedema and infection/Close-up

This picture shows a better view of the areas of early breakdown. There is redness, swelling and blistering. This is a medical emergency and the patient should be hospitalized for treatment of the cellulitis.

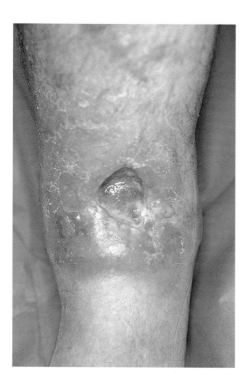

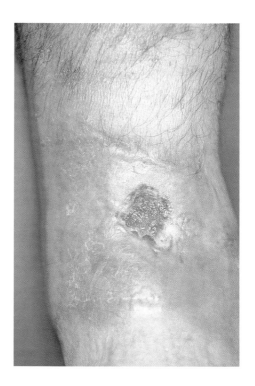

Figure 5.53a
Injury and lymphatic ulcer

Some cases of lymphatic obstruction start
with trauma. In this case, an automobile
accident caused a fracture of the tibia and
subsequent ulceration and chronic swelling
of the anterior portion of the leg. The
redness around the ulcer represents an
infection. The ulcer bed shows a yellow
exudate. He improved while hospitalized and
receiving systemic antibiotics. We think that
the improvement patients get from being
hospitalized is more than just due to the use
of intravenous antibiotics. Hospitalization
allows patients to rest and keep their legs
elevated, and puts the physician in charge of
the situation. For example, the use of topical
agents can be controlled.

Figure 5.53b
Injury and lymphatic ulcer/Healing

The infection was treated and the patient
was followed in the outpatient setting. Foam
dressings were used to provide absorbancy
and protection for the ulcer. The picture
shows less redness and swelling. The ulcer is
healing.

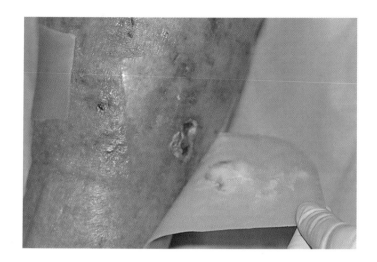

Figure 5.54
Debridement with occlusive dressings

This is now a well-established property of occlusive dressings. In many cases, occlusive dressings are able to stimulate painless debridement of the wounds. Here hydrocolloid dressings are being used to cover ulcers that were previously necrotic. The hydrocolloid "melts" into the wound, and often produces a brown exudate that may be mistaken for infection.

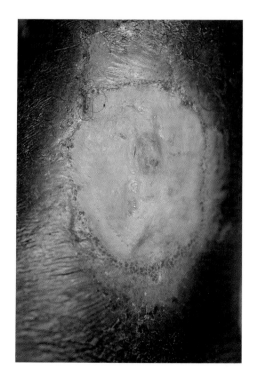

Figure 5.55a
Sickle cell ulcer

This 35-year-old man with sickle cell hemoglobinopathy has had persistent and excruciatingly painful ulceration on the medial aspect of his leg. The surrounding hyperpigmentation suggests venous disease, and many of these patients do have venous insufficiency. However, we have found that the clinical course of these sickle cell ulcers is different from that of venous ulcers. They are more painful, more resistant to treatment with compression and grafting, and can be deeper. They probably have a component of arteriolar disease. In some very resistant cases, we have combined split-thickness grafting with hyperbaric oxygen and transfusion with considerable success. At this stage the ulcer needs to be debrided.

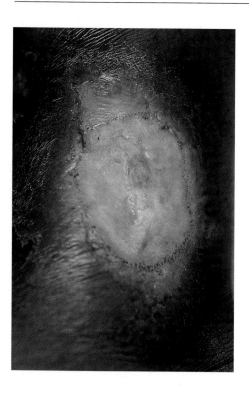

Figure 5.55b
Sickle cell ulcer/Close-up

The wound bed here in the larger ulcer is composed of a very tenacious necrotic material. Occlusive dressings were unable to debride it effectively and the patient required surgical debridement.

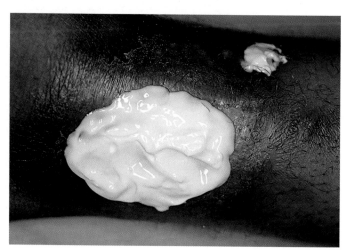

Figure 5.55c
Sickle cell ulcer/Debridement

We have often used the anesthetic EMLA to pretreat the ulcer before surgical debridement. This cream is kept in place for at least half an hour. Although on intact skin one generally uses EMLA under an occlusive film, this is not necessary with wounds.

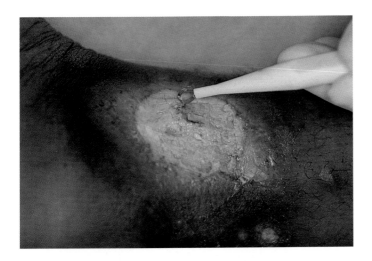

Figure 5.55d
Sickle cell ulcer/Debridement with a curette

Longitudinal and horizontal cuts are first made with a scalpel in the ulcer bed. This method basically divides the necrotic tissue into little squares which are more easily removable from the surrounding tissues. A curette is then used to remove the little squares.

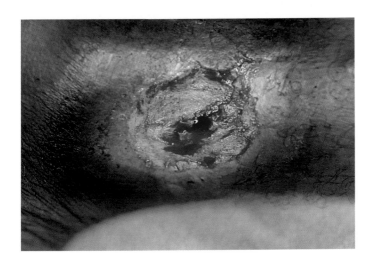

Figure 5.55e
Sickle cell ulcer/During debridement

Much of the yellow necrotic tissue has been removed. However, the ulcer bed contains very hard and fibrotic material. Regional or general anesthesia would be required to debride more extensively. However, so far the procedure has been painless. The wound was dressed with a hydrocolloid and with compression bandages.

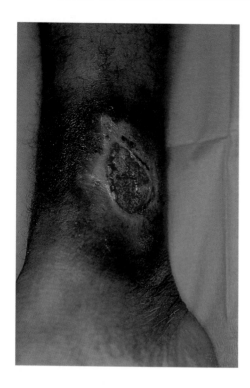

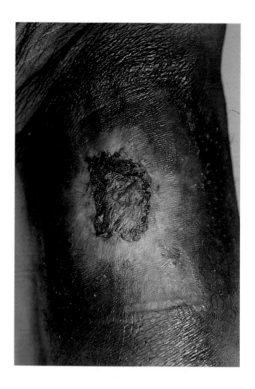

Figure 5.55f
Sickle cell ulcer/Healing

This picture was taken a few weeks later. There has been some healing from the edges of the ulcer. However, the improvement is not satisfactory and there is still considerable pain.

Figure 5.55g
Sickle cell ulcer/After grafting

Because healing was slow, the ulcer was debrided and grafted with a split-thickness autologous graft. This picture was taken 3 weeks after the grafting procedure and shows that most of the graft has taken. A foam dressing is being used at this time.

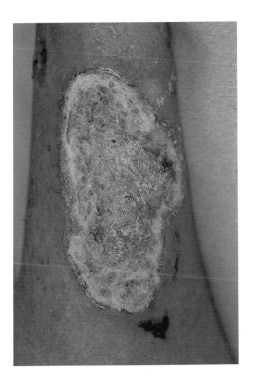

Figure 5.56a
Failed split-thickness graft

This 68-year-old woman with rheumatoid arthritis and multiple medical problems was quite a challenge. The ulcer, by its clinical features of undulating (scalloped) edges, is most likely a rheumatoid ulcer. However, several therapies failed, including the use of methotrexate. Compression therapy, in the hope that this may represent an unusual venous ulcer, also did not help. Histology from the ulcer's edge was non-specific but failed to show a vasculitis or obvious venous disease. Vascular studies showed venous insufficiency but good arterial flow. She was finally grafted but, as can be seen in this photograph, the graft became necrotic and most of it did not take.

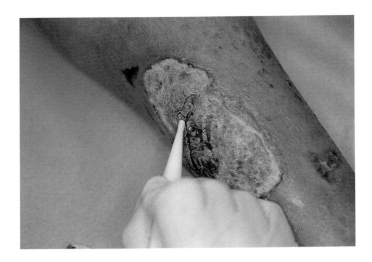

Figure 5.56b
Failed split-thickness graft/Debridement

It became necessary to remove the failed graft and debride the ulcer. The photograph shows the debridement being done with a curette.

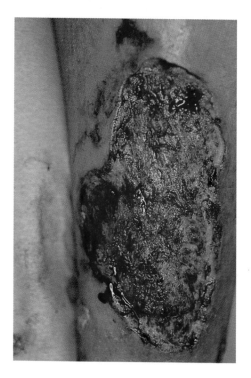

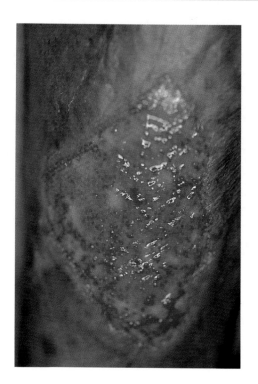

Figure 5.56c
Failed split-thickness graft/After debridement

The ulcer has been debrided rather extensively.

Figure 5.56d
Failed split-thickness graft/Healing

This picture was taken many weeks later and shows clear evidence of re-epithelialization. Debridement may have stimulated healing. It is also tempting to think that, even though grafting failed, the new skin may have somehow stimulated the healing process. We now recognize that grafts act as both tissue replacement and as "pharmacologic" agents capable of stimulating healing.

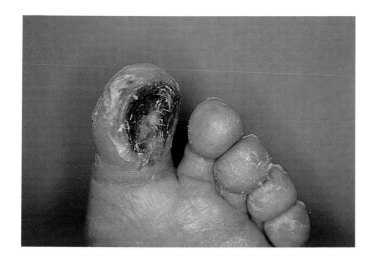

Figure 5.57a
Debridement of an arterial ulcer

This 70-year-old woman had inoperable arterial insufficiency, diabetes, and this non-healing ulcer of the big toe. She also had severe neuropathy and an insensate foot. The ulcer began after she stepped on a sewing needle that was stuck in her carpet. She repeatedly refused amputation, even when imaging studies suggested the possibility of osteomyelitis. Systemic antibiotics were used intravenously for 6 weeks, with some improvement. Here one sees substantial necrosis of the ulcer bed. There is also a yellow exudate in the center of the ulcer. No sinus tract was present and the underlying bone was not visible.

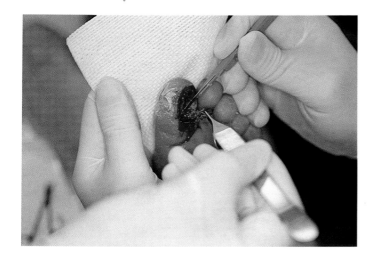

Figure 5.57b
Debridement of an arterial ulcer/Removal of necrotic tissue

After the application of EMLA cream and local anesthesia, a scalpel was used to remove the necrotic areas.

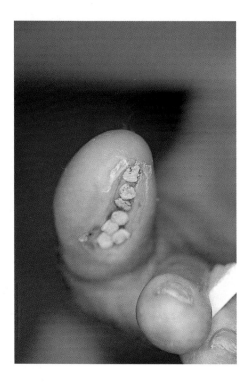

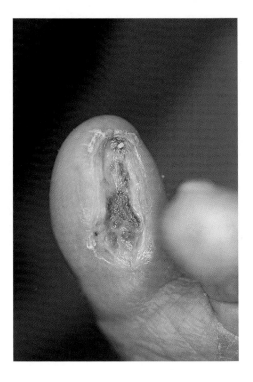

Figure 5.57c
Debridement of an arterial ulcer/Followed by pinch grafting

Right after the debridement, in the outpatient setting, a few pinches of skin from her abdomen were applied to the ulcer bed in the hope of stimulating healing.

Figure 5.57d
Debridement of an arterial ulcer/After pinch grafting

This photograph was taken a week later. The little pinches of skin have not taken and have fallen off. However, the "pharmacologic" action of the grafts may have stimulated ulcer healing. This approach is simple, cost-effective, and worth trying in difficult situations like this one.

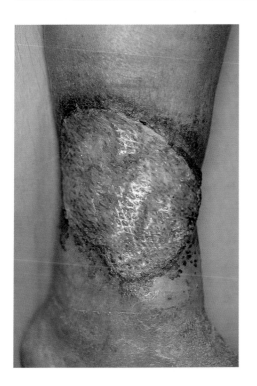

Figure 5.58
Meshed split-thickness graft

Of course, a more elegant and accepted way to graft ulcers is with meshed grafts. This large venous ulcer was grafted with an autologous split thickness graft meshed 1.5 to 1. The picture was taken 1 week after the surgical procedure, which was done in the hospital. Most of the graft seems to have taken and to be viable. Meshing is desirable when grafting these chronic wounds, or else the wound fluid accumulating beneath the graft will lift it off. Grafting is an under-utilized procedure for the management of non-healing or large ulcers. Although recurrence of the ulcer is not uncommon, the procedure provides patients with an ulcer-free interval of time and better quality of life.

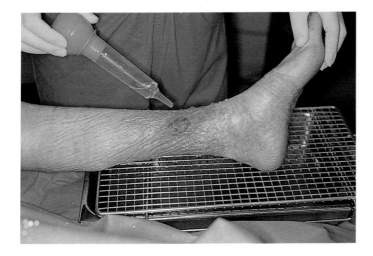

Figure 5.59
Wound irrigation

It is helpful to irrigate the wound extensively before debridement and grafting. This procedure may eliminate bacterial sheets and decrease bacterial burden. A useful device is a debridement tray, shown in this photograph. The tray collects all the saline, and the bottom pan has tubing connected to a suction pump. Using this tray, the ulcer can be irrigated with liters of saline in a convenient way.

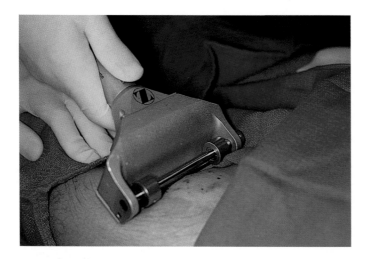

Figure 5.60a
Harvesting of split-thickness graft

The photograph shows the use of a dermatome to harvest a split-thickness graft from the anterior thigh. It is not a painless procedure and the skin has to be anesthetized first. One can, of course, use general anesthesia, but this carries more risks and may not be indicated when the graft to be harvested is small.

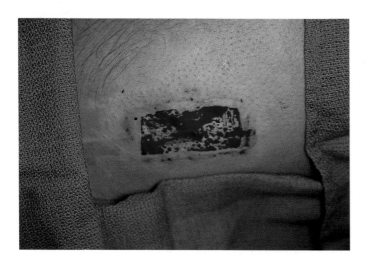

Figure 5.60b
Harvesting of split-thickness graft/Donor site

The wound created by harvesting a graft usually heals within 8–10 days, and the healing is accelerated if one uses an occlusive film. However, there are several problems associated with even a small donor site. The major problem is keeping the dressing in place if the patient is ambulatory. Movement of the thigh muscles tends to shift the dressing downward. In some cases, considerable pain is present.

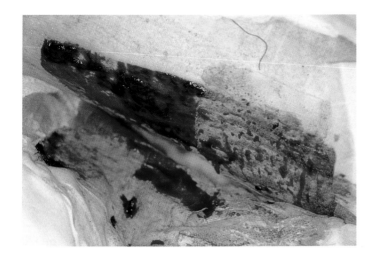

Figure 5.61
Large donor site

This 73-year-old woman has had metastatic melanoma of the skin over the last 2 years. These tumors have been managed with large excision and grafting. In this particular case, considerable donor tissue was needed. Here one sees the donor site on the lateral aspect of her thigh about 3 days after harvesting the graft. This donor site has been painful and she has required narcotics. A petrolatum-impregnated dressing has been used to create a moist wound environment.

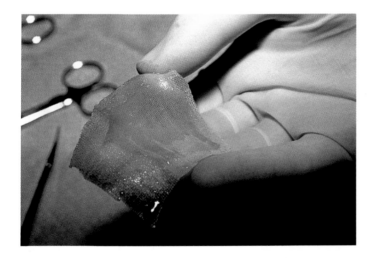

Figure 5.62
Cultured epithelial autograft

This cultured epithelium is dermal side up over a piece of petrolatum-impregnated gauze and is about to be applied over a venous ulcer. This type of cultured skin has now been used for about 15 years. It is very fragile and cannot be handled without first placing it on a gauze or dressing. Because it is an autograft, it was prepared from the patient's own skin and took several weeks to grow to this size. More recently, investigators have used similarly grown allografts to treat burns and chronic wounds.

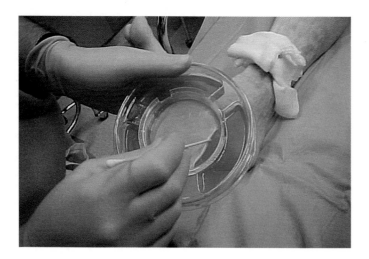

Figure 5.63a
Use of Graftskin

Recently, this type of bilayered skin construct has been available for the treatment of venous ulcers. It is composed of living keratinocytes and fibroblasts derived from neonatal foreskin. The keratinocyte sheet is grown over a type I bovine collagen gel that contains the fibroblasts. This product is delivered fresh and living in a transwell that contains special nutrients to keep the cells viable. Here, one sees the removal of Graftskin from the agar using the wooden end of a cotton applicator. It is about to be passed through a mesher before being applied to a venous ulcer.

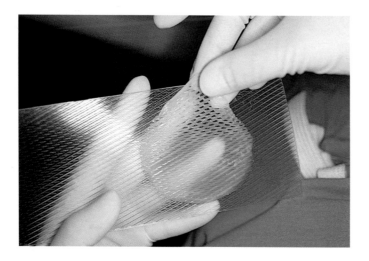

Figure 5.63b
Graftskin/Meshing

The cultured skin has been meshed at a ratio of 1.5 to 1. Here it is still on the adapter used to pass it through the mesher. It is not essential for Graftskin to be meshed. Fenestrations could be cut into the skin and still allow wound fluid to escape.

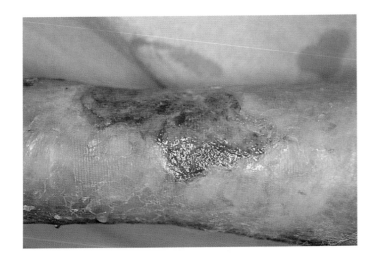

Figure 5.63c
Graftskin/Venous ulcer

This 92-year-old woman has had ulcers on and off for 30 years. It was decided to treat her ulcer with Graftskin, which has been found to be most helpful in ulcers of long duration. Although there has been some healing with a multi-layered elastic compression system, re-epithelialization has been very slow

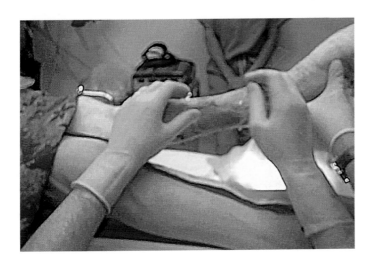

Figure 5.63d
Graftskin/Application

This photograph shows the patient's leg ulcer being treated with Graftskin. The meshed product was draped over the ulcer and stretched to cover most of the ulcer. No sutures are required, and the procedure is painless.

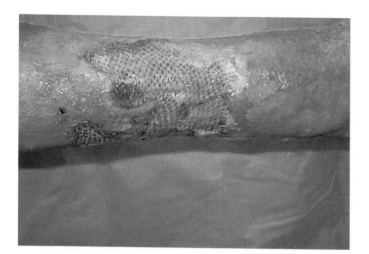

Figure 5.63e
Graftskin/In place

Here one sees the meshed
Graftskin over the circumferential
ulcer. Pain decreased dramatically.

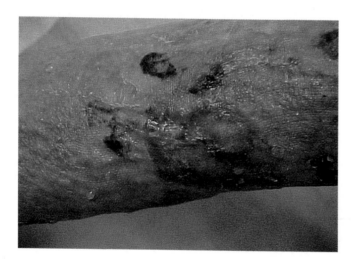

Figure 5.63f
Graftskin/After healing

Most of the ulcer healed with
Graftskin. This photograph was
taken 2 months after the
application.

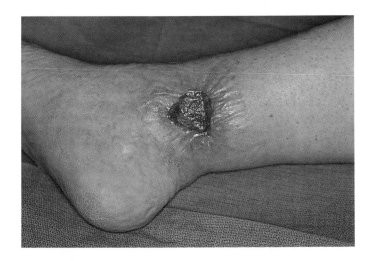

Figure 5.64a
Graftskin/Stimulation of healing

This woman in her 30s had a deep vein thrombosis and later developed a persistent venous ulcer. The wound is rather deep, and the ulcer bed appears pale. The edges are steep, as one sees in ulcers that are not healing.

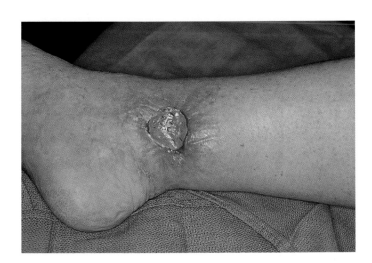

Figure 5.64b
Graftskin/Stimulation of healing

This photograph shows Graftskin in place. In this case, it was not meshed, but little cuts were made in it with a scalpel before application. These slits (0.5 to 1.0 cm in length) allow wound fluid to escape and thus prevent uplifting of Graftskin.

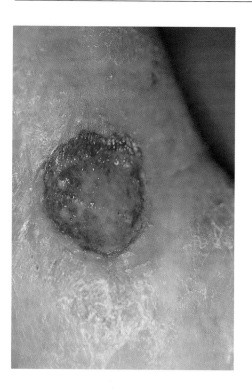

Figure 5.64c
Graftskin/Stimulation of healing

In some cases, one sees definite take of Graftskin and healing. In other cases, like this one, the Graftskin appears to stimulate the wound to heal. This photograph, taken 3 days after application, shows that the ulcer is now more shallow and that there is good granulation tissue. The yellow material represents hydrated Graftskin and, in some cases, can be mistaken for necrotic and infected tissue. Clinicians using Graftskin need to be aware of this phenomenon. One must not remove this material at this stage.

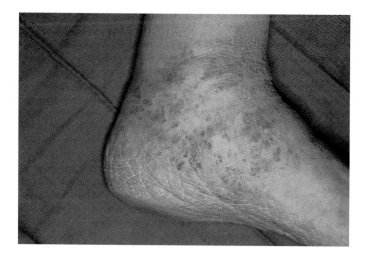

Figure 5.65
Failure to ulcerate

Eventually, one may come to the conclusion that venous insufficiency will inevitably result in ulceration. This, however, is not the case. This woman in her late 70s has had venous insufficiency for several decades and has refused to wear graded stockings, which she thinks are too uncomfortable. She has areas of atrophie blanche and many varicosities. Interestingly, the area has never ulcerated. There is no obvious lipodermatosclerosis, and that might explain her rather benign clinical course.

6 Inflammatory ulcers

Introduction

In this section we review a number of conditions which lead to chronic and often dramatic ulcerations. Excruciating pain is generally a hallmark of some of these ulcers. Proper diagnosis is essential here, because therapy is quite varied, depending on the underlying process. For example, ulcers due to cryofibrinogenemia respond well to the anabolic steroid stanozolol, cryoglobulinemia may be treated with interferons and immunosuppressive agents, and pyoderma gangrenosum responds dramatically to intravenous pulse steroid therapy and/or cyclosporin. Evaluation actually starts before we remove the bandages covering the wound and examine the wound itself. Indeed, the mental process leading to proper diagnosis and management starts as we are entering the examining room. We should look for signs of rheumatoid arthritis, for the typical features of scleroderma affecting the face and hands, and the cutaneous findings of lupus erythematosus. Hands affected by rheumatoid arthritis will tell us that the patient may have pyoderma gangrenosum or vasculitis. The malar rash of lupus erythematosus should lead us to expect the possibility of a wound associated with the presence of the antiphospholipid syndrome (lupus anticoagulant). We look for the Cushingoid appearance resulting from the chronic use of systemic corticosteroids, as wounds in these patients will typically have poor granulation tissue and respond to topical vitamin A compounds. A number of connective tissue disorders are associated with a livido pattern in the affected extremity; this clinical finding may be the result of dermal thrombi, cryofibrinogenemia, or cryoglobulinemia. Simply shaking the patient's hand will tell us about the possibility of scleroderma (indurated digits) or rheumatoid arthritis. Once we remove the bandages, we are able to determine whether the above clues are indeed valid. The appearance of pyoderma gangrenosum, with rolled purple borders and undermined edges, is typical. Ulcers due to the antiphospholipid syndrome have necrotic areas and are surrounded by areas of microlivedo, due to occlusion of small blood vessels. Location of the ulcers is also helpful. For example, erythema induratum, which has been associated with systemic tuberculous infection, commonly presents on the calf. The intensely painful ulcers due to thrombocytosis or treatment with hydroxyurea are generally on or around the malleoli. These and other clues can be of great help, before any laboratory tests or biopsies.

Biopsies are often of great help in the evaluation of this group of disorders. The biopsy site has to be chosen carefully. We generally biopsy the edge of the ulcer, and would choose skin immediately adjacent to necrotic areas. Histology may confirm the presence of dermal fibrin thrombi, and hence lead us in the direction of microthrombotic ulcers (cryofibrinogenemia, the antiphospholipid syndrome, cholesterol embolization). A mild inflammatory component around the occluded dermal vessels is seen in ulcers due to the antiphospholipid syndrome. The diagnosis of pyoderma gangrenosum, although based for the most part on clinical features, is also helped by histologic evaluation; histology will exclude an infectious process and will at least be consistent with pyoderma gangrenosum (i.e. a neutrophilic infiltrate and no vasculitis). Biopsies should be taken down to the subcutaneous tissue, so as not to miss the chance of diagnosing medium-sized vessel vasculitis (e.g. polyarteritis nodosa).

It will be noted that there is some overlap between this section and the previous one on vascular ulcers. This is because ulcers are often complicated by an inflammatory component, even though the etiology and pathogenesis are primarily related to occlusion of arteries or venous insufficiency. An obvious example of this is atrophie blanche. This painful condition is associated with vasculitis, arterial as well as venous disease, and, some clinicians even regard it as an entity in itself. In our experience, atrophie blanche tends to respond to high doses of pentoxifylline, sometimes in combination with colchicine. Lividoid vasculitis refers to an idiopathic condition where dermal blood vessels are occluded. Cholesterol embolization is another example where there can be a substantial inflammatory component even though the primary process is occlusion of small dermal and subcutaneous vessels by cholesterol crystals.

Clinical points

- Lipodermatosclerosis probably represents a spectrum of disease, ranging from an acute and intensely painful panniculitis to a more chronic and rather painless form associated with more established signs of venous insufficiency.
- The anabolic steroid stanozolol can provide dramatic clinical improvement and pain control to patients with lipodermatosclerosis.
- The differentiation between dermatitis and cellulitis of the leg is often difficult. It is often necessary to treat with systemic antibiotics.
- Skin grafting should be tried as therapy for inflammatory ulcers, such as erosive lichen planus or necrobiosis lipoidica diabeticorum. Pain control is often very dramatic after grafting.
- Some ulcers of the lower leg have clinical features of both pyoderma gangrenosum and necrobiosis lipoidica diabeticorum.
- Cyclosporin is a very effective therapeutic agent for pyoderma gangrenosum.
- Ulcers of erythema induratum (nodular vasculitis) are often on the calf.
- Calcinosis has no recognized effective treatment. Low-dose warfarin and calcium channel blockers may be worth trying.
- Calciphylaxis is often associated with renal disease and high mortality.
- Cutaneous injections of pentazocine can lead to severely fibrotic skin changes.
- Microlivedo refers to an incomplete pattern of lacy hyperpigmentation. This feature is common in ulcers due to occlusion of dermal vessels (microthrombotic ulcers).
- Ulcers caused by cryofibrinogenemia often respond dramatically to treatment with stanozolol.
- Cryoglobulinemia and ulceration is often associated with hepatitis C infection.
- Intravenous pulse steroid therapy can be an extremely effective and rapid treatment for pyoderma gangrenosum
- Cutaneous ulcers in patients with collagen vascular diseases often have unusual shapes and can mistakenly be thought to be factitial.
- In patients with systemic sclerosis (scleroderma), distal digital ulcers are usually due primarily to ischemia, while those on the metacarpal phalangeal joints are more likely the result of trauma.

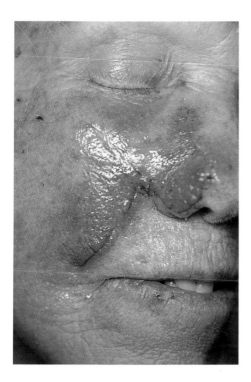

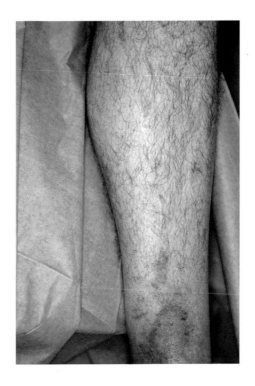

Figure 6.1
Contact dermatitis after surgery

This patient had a basal cell carcinoma removed from her cheek and the defect was repaired with a flap. After having used topical bacitracin ointment for several days, she returned with the involved area being red and slightly warm. There was no fever, tenderness, or pus. We thought that most likely she had a contact dermatitis. However, in spite of the absence of key clinical findings, we could not exclude a concomitant infection. Therefore, as is commonly done, she was treated with systemic antibiotics and the topical agent was stopped. The problem resolved within a few days.

Figure 6.2
Dermatitis after saphenous vein harvesting

This middle-aged man had a cardiac bypass operation for which the saphenous vein was harvested. A few months later, he developed this persistent dermatitis along the course of the incision and in the medial aspect of the leg. Dermatitis after harvesting of the saphenous vein is a reported complication of this procedure. Avoidance of topical agents, which could be sensitizing and aggravate the dermatitis, is important. Graded compression stockings are the treatment of choice.

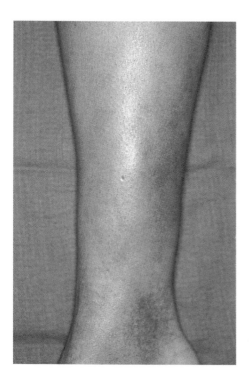

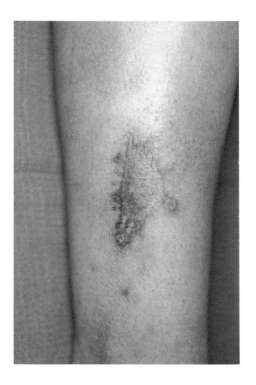

Figure 6.3a
Unusual case of lipodermatosclerosis (LDS)

LDS is commonly associated with venous insufficiency. It is actually a sclerosing panniculitis which results in fibrosis of the skin and subcutaneous tissues. The acute form of LDS can be very painful, while the chronic form is generally painless. There is probably a clinical spectrum between the acute and chronic form. This middle-aged woman seems to have both acute and chronic features of LDS. Here one sees on the medial aspect of the leg the swelling and mild hyperpigmentation that are more indicative of the acute phase.

Figure 6.3b
Unusual case of LDS/Hyperpigmentation

On the lateral aspect of the leg she had a hyperpigmented patch which is unusual for its location (lateral) and for the striking geometric configuration. There was no history of trauma. A biopsy did not show any evidence of Kaposi's sarcoma, which would be highly unusual in a woman but should be considered when there is localized hyperpigmentation on the lower leg. The treatment of LDS is compression stockings. If these are not well tolerated, the anabolic steroid stanozolol has been found to improve the condition.

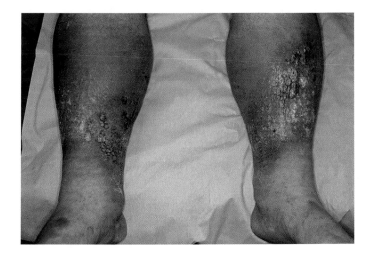

Figure 6.4
Bilateral venous dermatitis

A rather dramatic example of chronic dermatitis associated with venous insufficiency is shown in this photograph. There is redness, scaling, hyperpigmentation, and the typical "inverted bowling pin" or "champagne bottle" appearance of the legs, which are typical features of venous disease. In addition, there is a verrucous appearance of the skin, which suggests concomitant lymphatic disease. These patients are difficult to manage, and they often have a chronic cellulitis, perhaps because of the lymphatic obstruction. Hospitalization to treat the infection is frequent. Sometimes, systemic antibiotics (i.e. penicillin) need to be used on a chronic basis to control the infection.

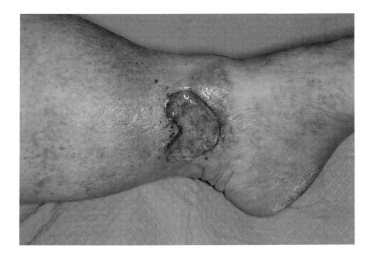

Figure 6.5a
Dermatitis and infection

This is a common combination in patients with venous ulcers, and it is necessary to address both conditions. The wound is debrided and systemic antibiotics are administered. We prefer to treat the dermatitis by avoiding all topical agents, including topical steroids, which could have ingredients that make the dermatitis worse. Gel dressings can be very helpful and soothing. On occasion, after treatment of the infection, we have used systemic corticosteroids for 2–3 weeks to get the dermatitis under control.

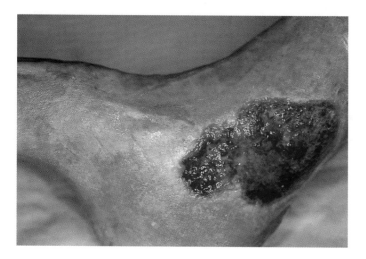

Figure 6.5b
Dermatitis and infection/Another case

Here too there is both a cellulitis and a dermatitis. The dermatitis appears to be in the dependent portion of the foot, a feature we have often associated with retention of fluid by the primary dressing. The reasons for this remain unclear. When we have collected wound fluid from an ulcer and applied it to the patient's own normal forearm skin (as in a patch test), we have been unable to elicit a reaction at that site. The granulation tissue here looks exuberant and has areas of necrosis; the ulcer bed is most likely infected.

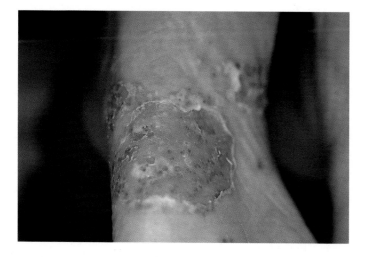

Figure 6.6
Pustular psoriasis and ulceration

Pustular psoriasis can be a life-threatening condition and is often associated with severe constitutional symptoms. Infection needs to be excluded in all cases, because the pustules of generalized infection with *Staphylococcus aureus* and herpes simplex can mimic the condition. As is often the case, the lesions are worse on the palms and soles. The photograph shows a plantar ulceration with surrounding pustules. Systemic agents (retinoids, methotrexate) are often used to treat severe pustular psoriasis. Occasionally, pustular psoriasis develops in patients with plaque psoriasis who have been treated with systemic steroids.

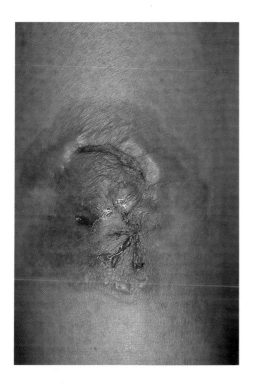

Figure 6.7
Erythema multiforme

Multiple blisters developed in this 34-year-old woman with recurrent erythema multiforme. These local inflammatory lesions are associated with recurrent oral or genital infection with herpes simplex. Treatment with antiviral agents can be helpful.

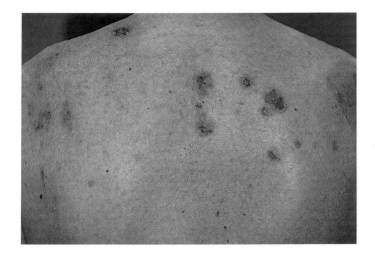

Figure 6.8a
Pemphigus vulgaris

This life-threatening blistering disorder generally involves the oral mucosa and, not uncommonly, the skin as well. It is an immunologic disorder associated with autoantibodies against structural proteins in the skin. The erosions seen in this photograph look mild and easy to heal. However, they can persist for months. Oral erosion and ulcers often require treatment with high doses of systemic corticosteroids.

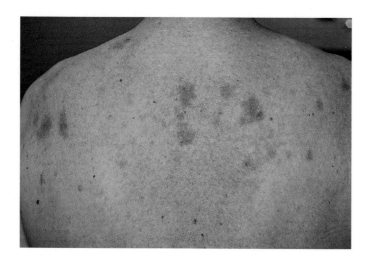

Figure 6.8b
Pemphigus vulgaris/Healed erosions

The erosions healed with systemic corticosteroids. An adherent foam dressing was used for wound care.

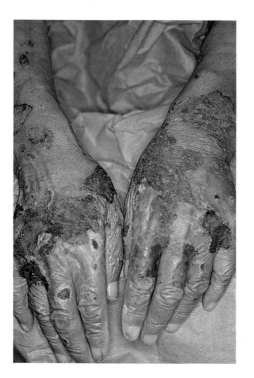

Figure 6.9
Bullous pemphigoid

Tense blisters developed on the arms and trunk of this elderly man. By direct immunofluorescence, the skin adjacent to the lesions had linear deposition of IgG and C3. The diagnosis of bullous pemphigoid was made. This condition is more common in the elderly. As in pemphigus, the treatment of bullous pemphigoid generally requires the use of systemic corticosteroids. Another condition, epidermolysis bullosa aquisita, can mimic bullous pemphigoid, but there are ways to distinguish the two. When painful, these erosions are best treated with a non-adherent gel dressing.

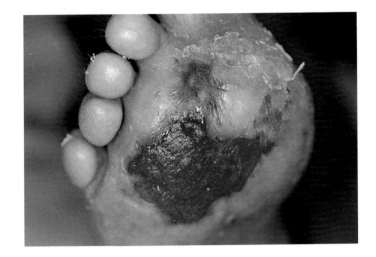

Figure 6.10a
Erosive lichen planus

Lichen planus is an inflammatory condition occurring in the oral and genital mucosa exclusively or as a widespread eruption of the skin. Rarely, it involves mainly the palms and soles. It can present as an overlap of lichen planus and lupus erythematosus of the palm and soles. In this particular patient, there was clear histologic evidence of lichen planus of the plantar surface. Occlusive wound dressings and intralesional injections of corticosteroids provided no relief from pain, and there was ongoing breakdown of the involved skin.

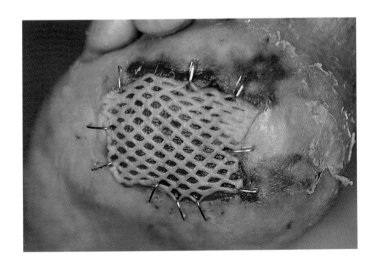

Figure 6.10b
Erosive lichen planus/Grafted

Clinicians do not use grafting often as a means of healing ulceration due to inflammatory processes. However, in selected situations, split-thickness autologous skin grafting (as in this case) can be very valuable in healing the ulcerations or, at the very least, stimulate healing. It is now recognized that grafts can not only provide new cells for the non-healing wound, but also stimulate endogenous healing.

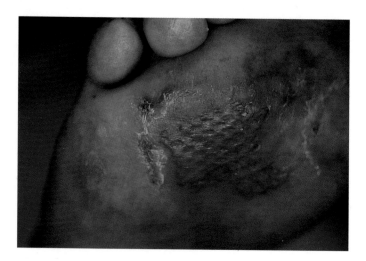

Figure 6.10c
Erosive lichen planus/Grafted

This photograph was taken 4 weeks after grafting. There is complete healing. Satellite lesions of lichen planus are still visible at the edges, however.

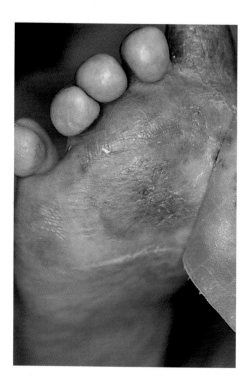

Figure 6.10d
Erosive lichen planus/Grafted

Several weeks later, the area has remained healed and is beginning to look more like normal skin. There seems to be much less of an inflammatory process, perhaps also as a result of treatment with a hydrocolloid dressing. This case illustrates very dramatically the potential of treating inflammatory conditions with grafts. One may at first make the assumption that such treatment should not work, because the underlying condition still exists. However, we think that the graft is altering (or conditioning) the microenvironment of the ulceration and the overall process.

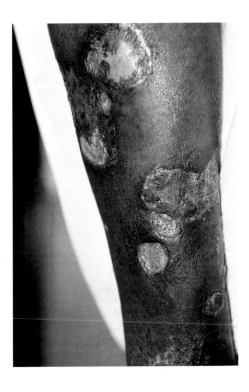

Figure 6.11
Sarcoidosis

It is not common for the granulomatous cutaneous lesions of sarcoidosis to ulcerate. This 38-year-old woman had approximately 30 areas of ulcerations on her lower legs. A biopsy showed non-caseating granulomas consistent with sarcoidosis. There was liver and lung involvement. She was treated with oral prednisone and plaquenyl. Eventually, the non-healing ulcers responded to treatment with cultured epidermal allografts. Bioengineered skin may be a promising treatment for inflammatory ulcers.

Figure 6.12a
Necrobiosis lipoidica diabeticorum (NLD)

NLD commonly ulcerates, as shown here in this woman with diabetes mellitus. NLD is a rather specific marker for diabetes. It develops in patients who have diabetes, or who will develop diabetes, or who have a strong family history of diabetes. The tibial location is typical, as is the yellow–orange color. Occasionally, NLD can resemble pyoderma gangrenosum. NLD ulcerations are difficult to treat. There have been reports of the successful use of autologous split-thickness grafts. Nicotinamide has been reported to be helpful. Occlusive dressings, for example hydrocolloids, can accelerate healing and protect this area, which is highly susceptible to trauma.

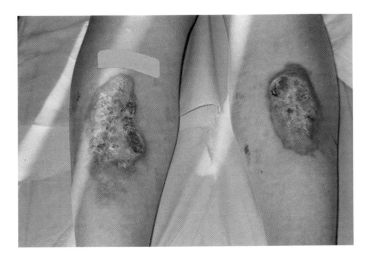

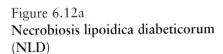

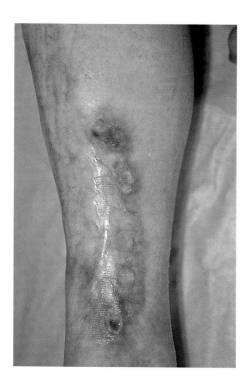

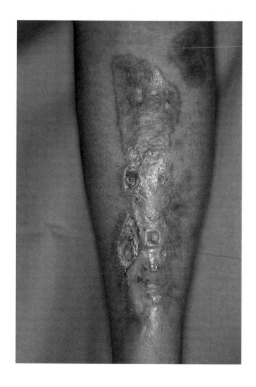

Figure 6.12b
**Necrobiosis lipoidica diabeticorum
(NLD)/Small punched-out ulcers**

This woman with insulin-dependent diabetes
presented with bilateral atrophic plaques
over both shins. These were yellowish in
color, had telangiectasia and became
ulcerated at the periphery. Biopsy confirmed
the diagnosis of NLD. If the ulcerations are
small, as in this patient, they can be managed
with intralesional corticosteroid injection,
but this is not always helpful.

Figure 6.12c
**Necrobiosis lipoidica diabeticorum
(NLD)/Recurrent**

Ulcerations often recur within NLD, as in
this case. She responded initially to
intralesional corticosteroid injections. In
some cases, we have treated patients with
systemic anti-inflammatory agents, such as
methotrexate or cyclosporin.

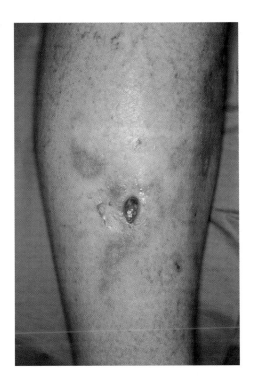

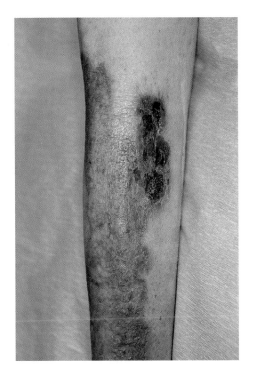

Figure 6.12d
Necrobiosis lipoidica diabeticorum (NLD)/Healing ulcer

This patient has had NLD for many years. Biopsies have confirmed this diagnosis. However, some of the histologic features have also been consistent with granuloma annulare. The histologic, and sometimes clinical, overlap between NLD and granuloma annulare are well known. The ulcers are presently healing with a hydrocolloid and high doses (800 mg three times a day) of pentoxifylline.

Figure 6.13
Necrobiosis lipoidica diabeticorum (NLD)/Pyoderma gangrenosum

We have had a number of patients with tibial lesions and ulcerations resembling NLD but with clinical features also suggestive of pyoderma gangrenosum. This elderly woman with many medical problems, including diabetes, is an example of this clinical presentation. Intralesional corticosteroid injections would heal the injected areas, but new lesions (see the necrotic dark areas) would develop next to it. Potent corticosteroids under occlusion seemed to help the situation for a period of time and prevent further ulcerations from developing.

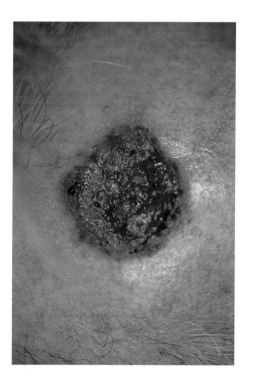

Figure 6.14
Pyoderma gangrenosum (PG)

The purple edges, the raised border, and the attempts at re-epithelialization within the ulcer bed, are extremely suggestive of PG. This man did not have associated diseases like rheumatoid arthritis, inflammatory bowel disease, leukemia, multiple myeloma, Behcet's disease or IgA gammopathy.

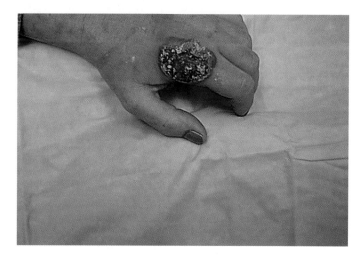

Figure 6.15
Pyoderma gangrenosum (PG) presenting with blisters

Initial lesions can start as blisters, which is a time when intralesional corticosteroids can help. This woman had a number of medical problems, including inflammatory bowel disease. The clinical course of the systemic problem often parallels that of PG. Cyclosporin has been a major breakthrough in the treatment of PG. We generally use it at a dose of 2.5–5 mg/kg and taper the dose slowly over a few weeks once the ulcer has healed.

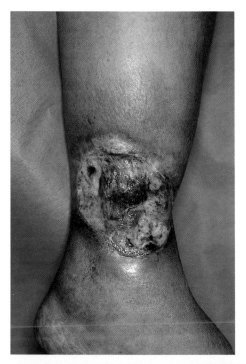

Figure 6.16a
Pyoderma gangrenosum (PG) with massive necrosis

As the name of the condition often implies, massive necrosis and gangrene can develop. It is not unusual for these patients to be debrided very extensively by clinicians who are not aware of the diagnosis. The problem with extensive debridement is that it can dramatically worsen the ulceration by the process of pathergy. This woman had rheumatoid arthritis and developed this ulceration within a period of a few weeks.

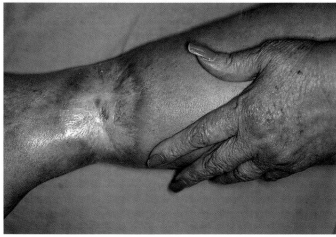

Figure 6.16b
Pyoderma gangrenosum (PG) with massive necrosis/Follow-up

The patient was treated with cyclosporin (5 mg/kg) and healed after several months. The appearance of the hand is suggestive of rheumatoid arthritis. Although cyclosporin is highly effective, it usually requires many weeks of treatment when used in these low but safer doses. If the serum creatinine increases or if hypertension develops, one needs to lower the dose for a period of time. Close monitoring of serum creatinine and blood pressure is required. There have been some reports of the successful use of topically applied cyclosporin, but this would only be applicable to the treatment of early and shallow ulcers.

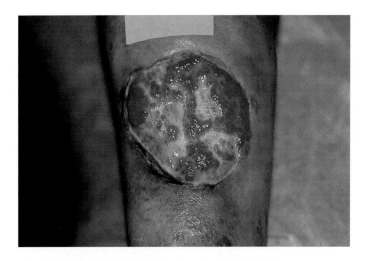

Figure 6.17
Pyoderma gangrenosum (PG) during treatment

This 45-year-old man presented with multiple rapidly enlarging ulcers with a violaceous and undermined border characteristic of PG. No associated systemic involvement could be found. The condition improved with large doses of systemic corticosteroids. In general, oral prednisone at a dose of at least 60 mg/day is required for initial treatment.

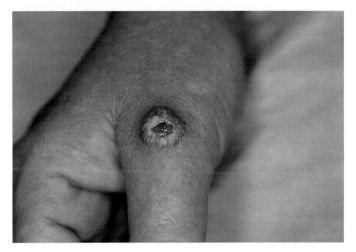

Figure 6.18a
Pyoderma gangrenosum (PG) and intralesional corticosteroids

This woman is in her late 40s and has no disease associated with PG. She develops recurrent blisters, and these result in ulcers with purple edges and undermined borders. This photograph shows a typical blister, days after its initial appearance.

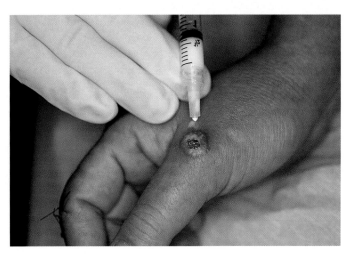

Figure 6.18b
Pyoderma gangrenosum (PG) and intralesional corticosteroids/Injection

The photograph shows the lesion being injected with 20 mg/ml of triamcinolone acetonide.

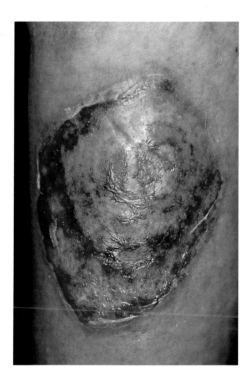

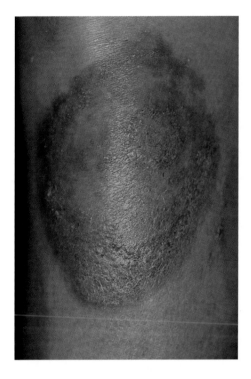

Figure 6.19a
Pyoderma gangrenosum (PG) and purple edges

This clinical feature is particularly evident in this 44-year-old woman with idiopathic PG. For a while, she was thought to have had a brown recluse spider bite, but the diagnosis of PG was made on clinical grounds and the histology was consistent with it. It should be noted that the diagnosis of PG is mainly clinical and that histologic results (i.e. neutrophilic infiltration or granulomatous variant) are only suggestive. Cultures for mycobacteria and fungi are often required during the evaluation process.

Figure 6. 19b
Pyoderma gangrenosum (PG) and purple edges/Follow-up

This patient was treated and healed after a 4-day course of intravenous pulse steroid therapy. This picture was taken 1 week later. During her hospital course, each day she received 1 g of methylprednisolone, with careful attention to serum electrolytes and cardiac rhythm. Patients on diuretics are more susceptible to electrolyte shifts during treatment with massive doses of corticosteroids, and arrythmias can develop in that setting. In such patients, telemetry may be necessary or treatment with alternative therapies (i.e. cyclosporin) would be preferable.

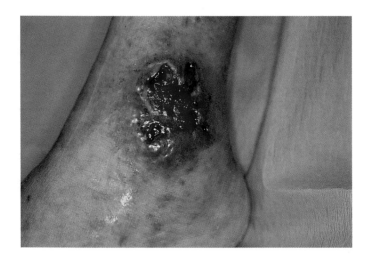

Figure 6.20
Pyoderma gangrenosum (PG)-like in a child

The patient was seen at multiple medical centers for Wiskott–Aldrich syndrome. Apparently, this ulceration developed after treatment with intravenous immunoglobulin. Clinically, the ulcer is most consistent with PG, although cutaneous lymphoma should be considered. Histology of a biopsy specimen showed a lymphocytic vasculitis with fibrinoid necrosis consistent with livedo vasculitis. The ulcer healed after discontinuing immunoglobulin therapy and with local care with a hydrocolloid dressing and leg compression.

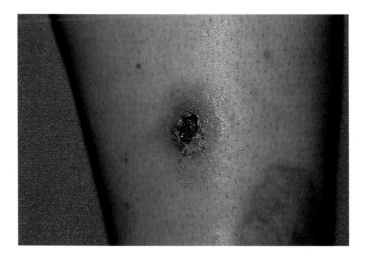

Figure 6.21
Pyoderma gangrenosum (PG) and Behcet's disease

This patient had incapacitating arthritis and oral and genital ulcers. Skin ulcers had developed and healed in the past, as shown by the scar in the photograph. The small ulceration seen here shows the classical purple edges of PG. She healed with intravenous pulse steroid therapy.

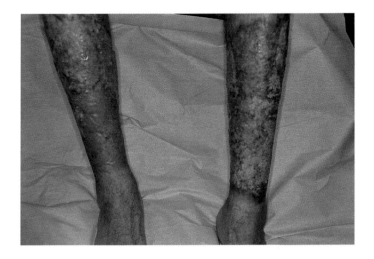

Figure 6.22a
Pyoderma gangrenosum (PG) and Sweet's syndrome

The patient presented with extensive ulcers on both legs which began as bullous lesions 1 day after he received an intramuscular injection of penicillin. During his clinical course, the lesions evolved to what is seen in the photograph and he was thought to have PG. Biopsy of the ulcerations showed an intense neutrophilic infiltration which could be consistent with Sweet's syndrome or PG. Shortly thereafter, he was diagnosed as having a rare form of leukemia (chronic neutrophilic leukemia).

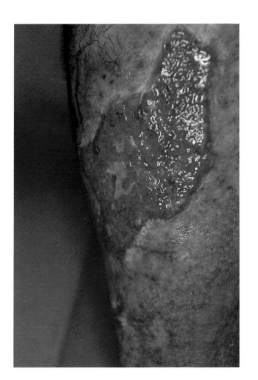

Figure 6.22b
Pyoderma gangrenosum (PG) and Sweet's syndrome/Follow-up

It is difficult to know whether this patient had Sweet's syndrome or PG, two conditions which can be associated with a myeloproliferative disorder. He was treated with a number of approaches, including systemic corticosteroids, cyclosporin, and chemotherapy for his leukemia. The most difficult problem was managing the wound pain, which was best done with hydrogels. This clinical photograph was taken while the ulceration was improving.

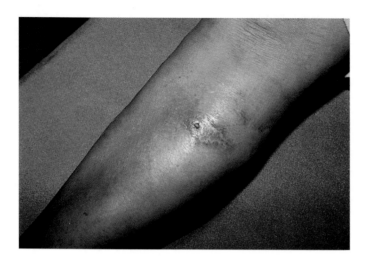

Figure 6.23
Erythema induratum

Ulcers of erythema induratum can look rather non-specific and are usually located on the calf. The condition is also called nodular vasculitis. Its association with systemic tuberculous infection is still the subject of considerable controversy. However, clinicians still tend to treat these patients with antituberculous drugs. This particular patient had a positive tuberculin test and has been improving on isoniazid.

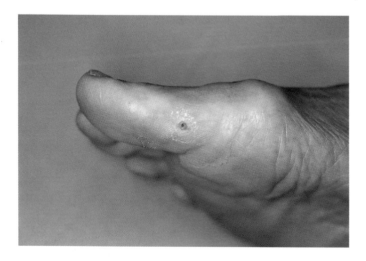

Figure 6.24
Calcinosis

This patient has systemic sclerosis (scleroderma) and a painful non-healing ulcer on the big toe. The ulcerated area was hard to the touch and was shown to contain calcium deposits. Patients with scleroderma commonly develop calcinosis, especially in the subgroup called CREST syndrome. In this case, an excision was performed to remove the calcified tissue.

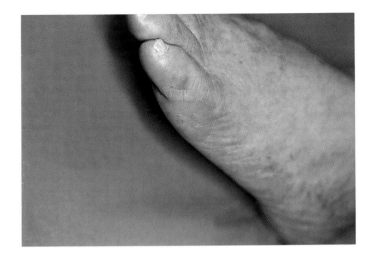

Figure 6.25
Calcinosis

In this other patient with systemic sclerosis (scleroderma), the calcium deposits presented as a clinically inflammatory area on the lateral portion of the foot. It was not possible to remove these areas surgically and she was treated with low doses of warfarin (2.5 mg/day), which have been reported to be helpful for calcinosis. The intent is not to alter the prothrombin time, but rather to keep it normal. The mechanisms by which warfarin works in some of these situations are not known. Another approach is to use a calcium channel blocker, such as diltiazam. However, large doses of this drug may be necessary.

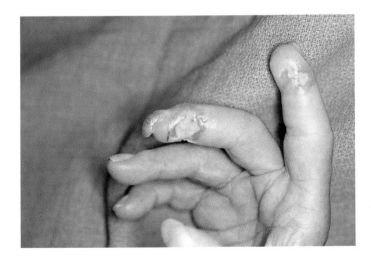

Figure 6.26
Digital ulcers

Patients with systemic sclerosis (scleroderma) often develop digital ulcerations. Those on the knuckles are often due to trauma in the setting of fibrotic skin. Those that are located more distally, like the ones shown here, are more likely to be the result of significant ischemia. It is important to recognize this distinction because vasodilators, if they work at all, would be most helpful in distal ulcers. This patient, however, did not respond to vasodilators. Periodic debridement and hyperbaric oxygen were tried, with marginal results. Calcinosis often complicates these ulcers and makes healing more difficult. Autoamputation is often the outcome.

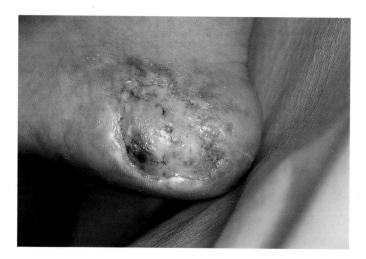

Figure 6.27
Inflammatory ulcer in systemic sclerosis (scleroderma)

When this patient was evaluated, considerable thought was given to the possibility of cryofibrino-genemia because of the necrotic areas and microlivedo pattern around the ulcer. However, her plasma was negative for cryofibrinogen and a biopsy did not show evidence of fibrin thrombi, which are common in cryofibrinogenemia. No vasculitis was present but there was some calcium deposition. The lesion was very painful. We treated her with a hydrocolloid to stimulate granulation tissue and for pain relief. We also treated her with warfarin. Her pain improved and she was able to ambulate with less discomfort.

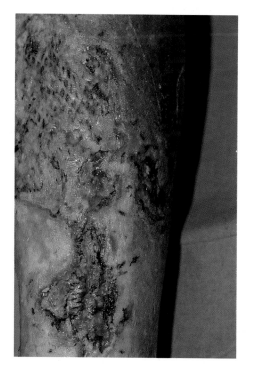

Figure 6.28a
Calcinosis and ulcers

This middle-aged woman had classical CREST syndrome, which represents a subgroup of patients with systemic sclerosis (scleroderma). Her main clinical problems were these extensive ulcerations on the lower extremities which were literally filled with calcium deposits. Various wound care approaches were tried with minimal results, including the use of hydrocolloids and hydrogels. The photograph shows the wound a week after split-thickness skin grafting. There was hope that this graft would take or stimulate the wound to heal.

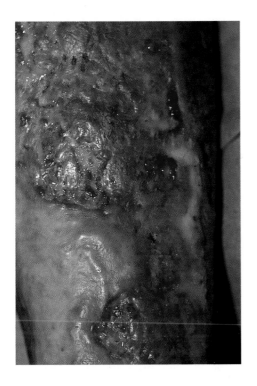

Figure 6.28b
Calcinosis and ulcers/Follow-up

The graft did seem to stimulate ulcer healing. Here one sees better granulation tissue and some re-epithelialization. After another few weeks, sudden worsening of the ulcer occurred and was associated with clinical signs of infection. However, the point here is that it may be worthwhile to graft some of these inflammatory ulcers. With the availability of bioengineered skin, it may be possible to do so in a non-invasive fashion and repeatedly.

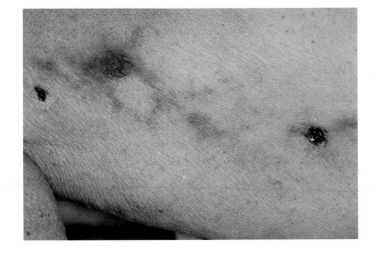

Figure 6.29
Calciphylaxis

This woman's thigh shows areas of livedo reticularis and necrotic skin. The clinical picture is highly suggestive of calciphylaxis, which represents deposition of calcium crystals in the wall of blood vessels. There is a high mortality associated with this presentation, as many patients have severe renal disease. In this particular patient, we tried the anabolic steroid stanozolol without significant improvement. There have since been reports in the literature about the successful use of calcium channel blockers.

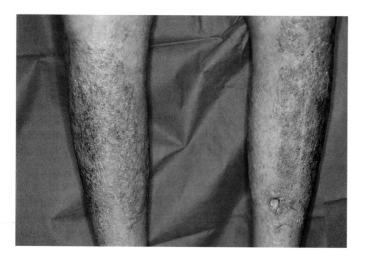

Figure 6.30a
Eosinophilic fasciitis (EF)

This elderly woman presented with classic features of eosinophilic fasciitis. She developed swelling of the lower extremities with characteristic sparing of the toes, peripheral blood eosinophilia, and muscle pain. In a matter of a few weeks, she had ankle contractures and extensive fibrosis of the involved skin. She had not taken L-tryptophan, which has been implicated in many of the cases of EF, but had been on nicotinic acid. Even though L-tryptophan has been taken off the market now, we still occasionally see new cases of EF. The photograph shows an ulceration within the very fibrotic skin. Such ulcers have proved to be difficult to heal. In addition, the skin was scaly and hyperpigmented, and we could not exclude the possibility of superimposed contact dermatitis.

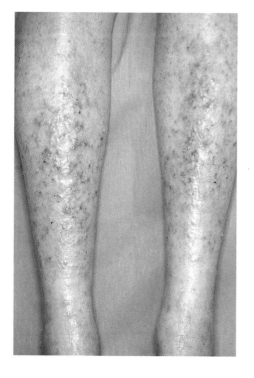

Figure 6.30b
Eosinophilic fasciitis (EF)/Follow-up

The patient was treated with a number of agents, including systemic corticosteroids (up to 50 mg/day), which are the drugs of choice for EF. The ulcer healed with this approach. Oral isotretinoin for a few weeks seems to have improved the dermatitic component. She required small doses of systemic corticosteroids, about 15–20 mg/day, to keep the fibrotic process and dermatitic component under control. Four years later, the fibrosis has diminished, and the ankle contractures have improved. However, periodically, the erosions and dermatitis one sees in this photograph recur and necessitate an increase in the dose of systemic corticosteroids.

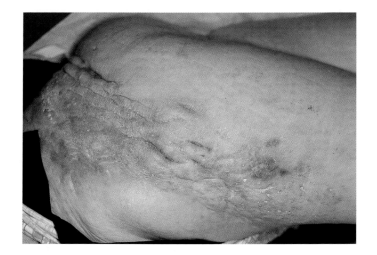

Figure 6.31a
Pentazocine-induced ulcers

This 52-year-old health-care professional used subcutaneous injections of pentazocine to relieve the pain of an unrelated condition. Over the next several years, she developed an extremely fibrotic reaction which encompassed most of her thighs and extended down to muscle. Ulcerations, sinus tracts and frequent infections were a major problem leading to numerous hospitalizations and chronic use of antibiotics. This is a well-recognized complication of pentazocine injections.

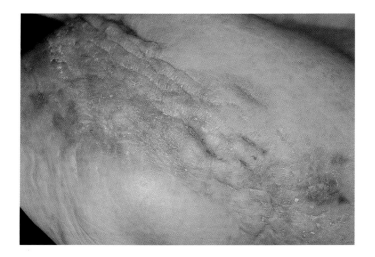

Figure 6.31b
Pentazocine-induced ulcers/Close-up

Here one can see some of the sinus tracts on the thigh. The fibrotic skin is thrown up into thick and hard folds. The patient would frequently become septic. We agreed with her surgeons that a drastic operation to remove all the diseased skin and sinus tracts would be necessary.

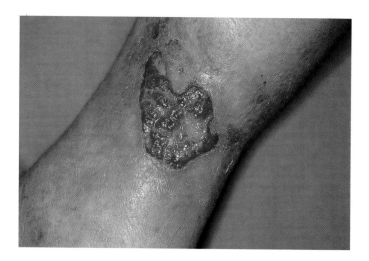

Figure 6.32a
Rheumatoid ulcer/No vasculitis

Ulcers developing in the setting of rheumatoid arthritis can be due to a number of causes, such as vasculitis, pyoderma gangrenosum, cryofibrinogenemia, cryoglobulinemia, and the antiphospholipid syndrome. Many ulcers, however, are difficult to classify. The one shown here falls into this category. There was no clinical or histologic evidence of vasculitis, and serum and blood studies failed to show cryoglobulins and cryofibrinogen, and anticardiolipin antibodies. We have found that many of these ulcers, like the one shown here, have an angular configuration or an undulating border. They prove difficult to treat, even with optimal wound care and potent systemic immunosuppressive agents.

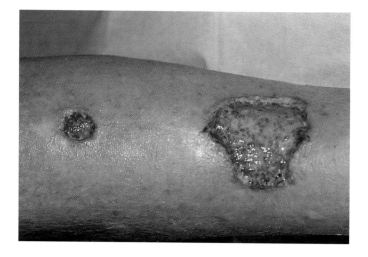

Figure 6.32b
Rheumatoid ulcer/Vasculitis

This 62-year-old woman had a long history of rheumatoid arthritis, which had been treated with systemic corticosteroids, plaquenyl, and methotrexate. She developed painful ulcers on her left leg. A biopsy showed histologic changes of vasculitis. Treatment with an increased dose of prednisone, with cyclophosphamide, and with the application of occlusive dressings, was successful in healing the ulcers over the course of 8 months.

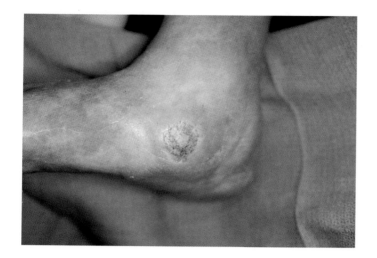

Figure 6.33
Rheumatoid ulcer and pressure

This wheelchair-bound elderly woman with incapacitating rheumatoid arthritis has had recurrent ulcers over the medial malleolus. She has severe knee and ankle deformities and has been on systemic corticosteroids for years. Because there was also very severe edema of the lower leg and non-healing rheumatoid ulcers on her calf, we applied a four-layer compression bandage from the toes to below the knee. The area around the ulcer was padded extensively with a wool wrap to fill in the concave areas around the malleolus and avoid excessive pressure over the ulcer. She would be a good candidate for a Scotch cast boot or a contact cast.

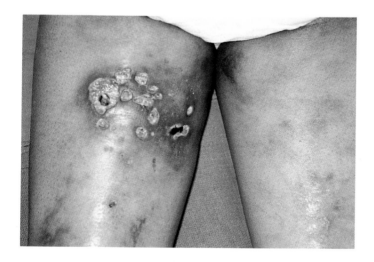

Figure 6.34a
Cutaneous lupus erythematosus

The involved skin is studded with necrotic and painful ulcers and is surrounded by areas of livedo. Clinically, these ulcers are consistent with a number of conditions, including pyoderma gangrenosum, panniculitis, and cryofibrinogenemia. She did have plasma cryofibrinogen, but the histology was most consistent with a panniculitis.

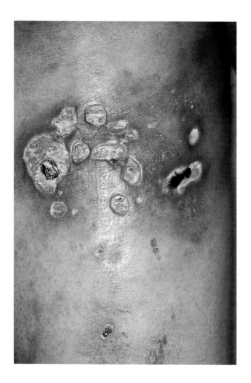

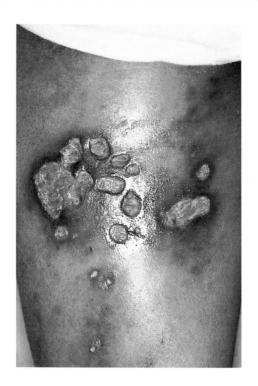

Figure 6.34b
Cutanenous lupus erythematosus/Close-up

This photograph shows the areas of necrosis and the microlivedo pattern.

Figure 6.34c
Cutaneous lupus erythematosus/After hydrocolloid

Pain management and debridement were the first considerations. The patient was treated with a hydrocolloid, which relieved the pain and painlessly debrided the ulcerations. With this treatment, there has been substantial improvement, with disappearance of the necrotic tissue and better granulation tissue. She will require systemic therapy to treat these ulcers, such as systemic corticosteroids or cyclosporin.

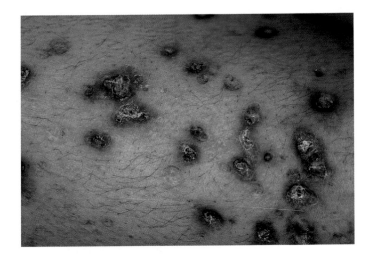

Figure 6.35
Lupus panniculitis

The patient has systemic lupus erythematosus and has developed numerous small ulcerations which are very painful. Biopsy showed a lobular panniculitis. She responded nicely to systemic corticosteroids. It is important not to dismiss such ulcers as factitial, even though their shape might suggest that possibility initially.

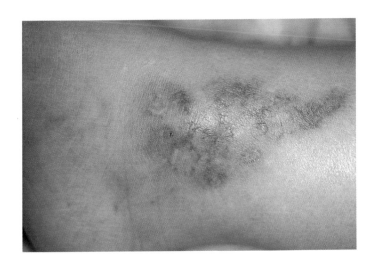

Figure 6.36
Livedo vasculitis

This middle-aged woman had very painful purple lesions on her lower leg. They would periodically ulcerate. Histologically, there were fibrin thrombi within dermal vessels. These thrombi can be seen in the setting of cryofibrinogenemia or the antiphospholipid syndrome. However, there was no plasma cryofibrinogen or anticardiolipin antibodies. The acute phase of this problem was treated successfully with the anabolic steroid stanozolol, which has fibrinolytic properties. She was also maintained on pentoxifylline. This clinical and histologic picture may be seen in a variety of conditions. The underlying, common finding is occlusion of small cutaneous vessels; we have called it "microthrombotic disease".

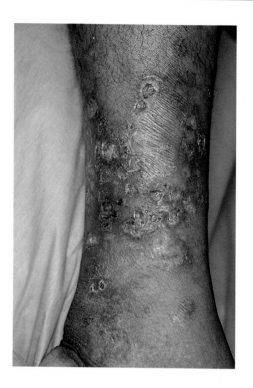

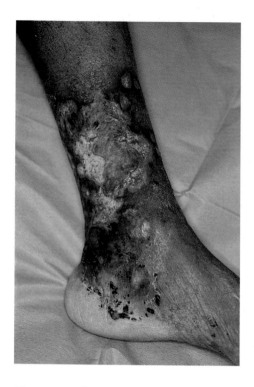

Figure 6.37a
Systemic periarteritis nodosa

This 61-year-old man has proven periarteritis nodosa with kidney involvement. He has been on methotrexate and other immunosuppressive agents. Complicating his clinical picture are these painful and recurrent ulcerations on his lower legs. New lesions would appear as purple areas and would show histologic evidence of leukocytoclastic vasculitis. Medium-sized vessels in his skin did not seem to be involved.

Figure 6.37b
Systemic periarteritis nodosa/New ulcerations

The purple areas would ulcerate and, in time, the patient would present with larger ulcers involving most of the lower leg. He was treated with a combination of methotrexate and cyclosporin but did not seem to respond well.

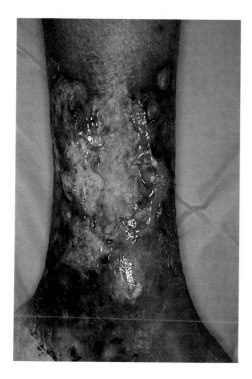

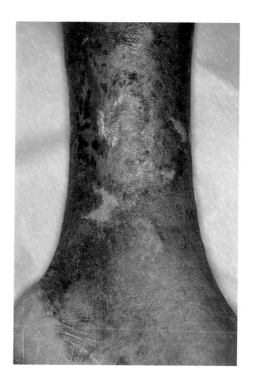

Figure 6.37c
Systemic periarteritis nodosa/Wound care

The patient was treated with a gel that promoted moist wound healing and helped in autolytic debridement. The photograph shows the gel in place. It was important to keep the wound from drying because the pain would worsen.

Figure 6.37d
Systemic periarteritis nodosa/Healed ulcers

The patient was kept on oral methotrexate. His ulcers seemed to improve after he was started on sulfamethoxazole for pneumocystis pneumonia (PCP) prophylaxis.

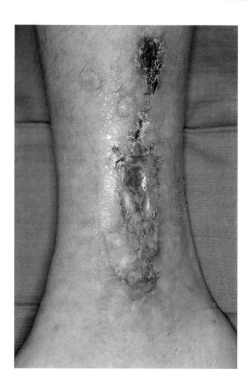

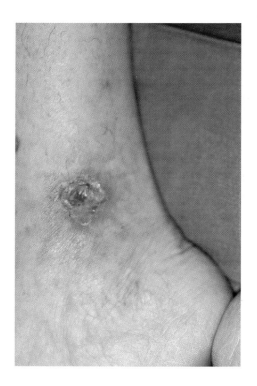

Figure 6.38a
Periarteritis nodosa

This patient had a long history of inflammatory bowel disease and leg ulcerations, which were thought to represent pyoderma gangrenosum. She improved dramatically on treatment with cyclosporin but worsened quickly when this drug was stopped because of concerns about her serum creatinine level. When we saw her, we were impressed by the necrotic appearance of some of these ulcers. An area at the border of the inferior ulcer was biopsied and showed classic findings for periarteritis nodosa, with destruction of medium-sized vessels.

Figure 6.38b
Periarteritis nodosa (opposite leg)

There was considerable heterogeneity in the appearance of this patient's ulcers. This one on the medial aspect of the other leg shows no necrosis and is in fact healing. There is a slight microlivedo pattern surrounding the ulcer.

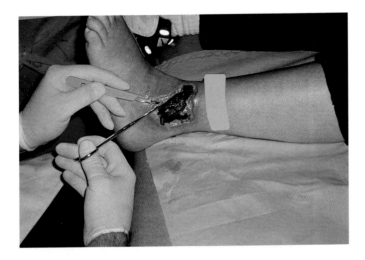

Figure 6.39a
Wegener's granulomatosis

The patient has an established diagnosis of Wegener's granulomatosis. These patients develop sinusitis, and pulmonary and renal involvement. They commonly have serum autoantibodies to c-ANCA. This large necrotic ulcer needed surgical debridement to accelerate healing.

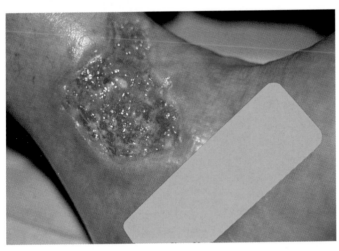

Figure 6.39b
Wegener's granulomatosis/After debridement

This photograph was taken about 3 weeks after the initial debridement. There is now good granulation tissue and some evidence of re-epithelialization.

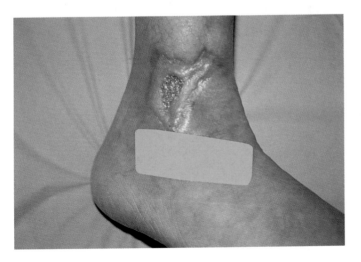

Figure 6.39c
Wegener's granulomatosis/Follow-up

Six weeks after the initial presentation, there has been considerable healing. The patient was kept on her systemic immunosuppressive therapy for Wegener's granulomatosis. This case illustrates the importance of following basic wound care principles in conditions that are inflammatory. We find that some clinicians often emphasize systemic therapy in these cases without proper attention to wound care.

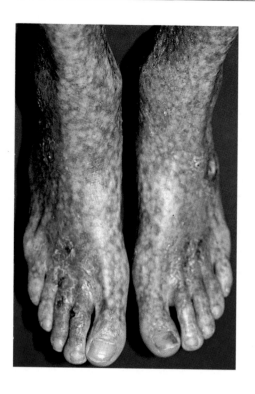

Figure 6.40a
Antiphospholipid syndrome

This belongs to the group of microthrombotic diseases, and is often associated with a lupus anticoagulant and anticardiolipin antibodies. It can cause severe systemic symptoms and spontaneous abortions. This Caucasian man with the antiphospholipid syndrome has extensive livedo reticularis and very painful ulcers.

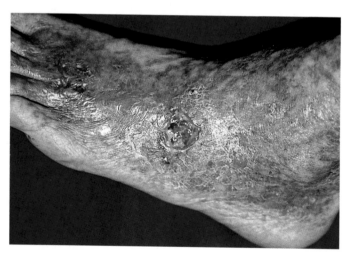

Figure 6.40b
Antiphospholipid syndrome/Ulcer

Biopsies of these ulcers will often show fibrin thrombi within dermal vessels with a slight perivascular lymphocytic infiltrate. In the past, we have found that these patients do not respond well to stanozolol, which is our drug of choice in the setting of fibrin thrombi and cryofibrinogenemia. This patient was treated wtih systemic immunosuppressive agents.

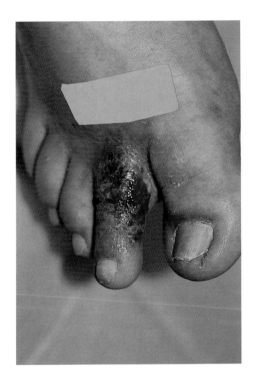

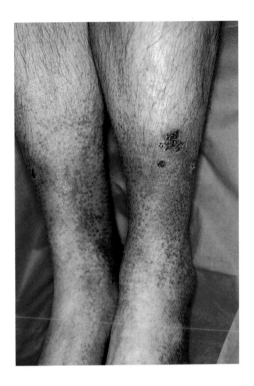

Figure 6.41
Antiphospholipid syndrome and systemic involvement

Many patients with this condition have systemic disease, and the present recommendation is to treat them with warfarin to prevent complications from clotting. This 20-year-old man had a history of myocardial infarction, deep vein thrombosis, and pulmonary embolism. A non-healing ulcer was present on his right second toe. Work-up showed high levels of anticardiolipin antibodies. Despite treatment with warfarin, the ulcer did not heal. He was treated with cultured epidermal allografts with complete closure within 10 days. Azathioprine, at a dose of 100 mg/day, was also used to treat his overall condition.

Figure 6.42a
Cryofibrinogenemia with widespread skin involvement

This 44-year-old man has purpura and ulcerations, with areas of livedo reticularis. When he was first seen, a number of diagnoses were considered. These included cryofibrinogenemia, cryoglobulinemia, vasculitis, Waldenstrom's macroglobulinemia, and the antiphospholipid syndrome. His plasma was positive for cryofibrinogen and biopsies of the purple areas showed fibrin thrombi within dermal blood vessels. This suggested that his cutaneous findings were most likely due to cyrofibrinogenemia.

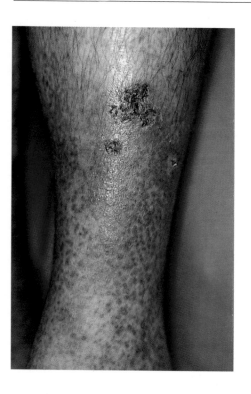

Figure 6.42b
Cryofibrinogenemia with widespread skin involvement/Close up

The crusted and necrotic appearance of the patient's ulcerations is more evident here. Pain was excruciating.

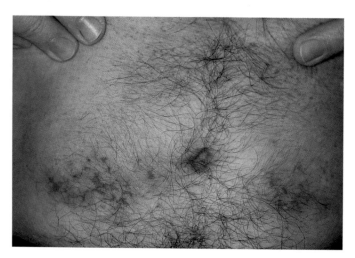

Figure 6.42c
Cryofibrinogenemia with widespread skin involvement/Chest

The patient had lesions elsewhere on his body, such as the ones shown here. They were angular in shape, a finding we have often observed in other inflammatory conditions and when small cutaneous blood vessels are occluded. He responded dramatically to the anabolic steroid stanozolol at a dose of 6 mg/day. Surprisingly, patients with cryofibrinogenemia do not consistently experience worsening of their symptoms upon cold exposure.

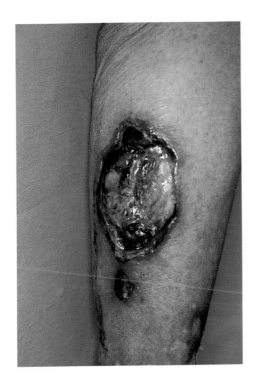

Figure 6.43
Cryofibrinogenemia

This dramatic ulceration developed within a few weeks in an 87-year-old man with many medical problems, including severe congestive heart failure. By plasma measurements and by histology, we made the diagnosis of cryofibrinogenemic ulceration. We wanted to give him stanozolol but this drug can cause substantial sodium retention and can greatly worsen congestive heart failure. We decided to hospitalize him and to treat him with stanozolol in a controlled setting where he could be closely monitored. His pain disappeared quickly and the ulcer ultimately healed with stanozolol.

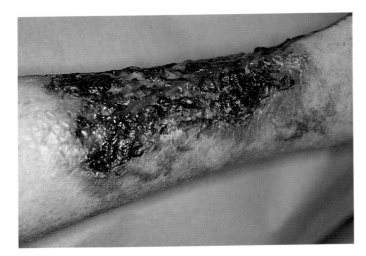

Figure 6.44
Cryoglobulinemia

The extensive necrosis and livedo pattern shown here should always raise the suspicion of ulcerations due to obstruction of small blood vessels. In this case, the underlying condition was cryoglobulinemia. However, a similar presentation would be seen with other conditions where microthrombi are seen in the dermis, i.e. cryofibrinogenemia, antiphospholipid syndrome. Patients such as this one often need therapy with immunosuppressive agents. Concomitant hepatitis C infection should always be excluded.

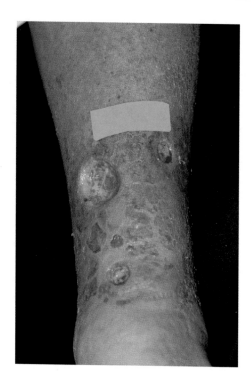

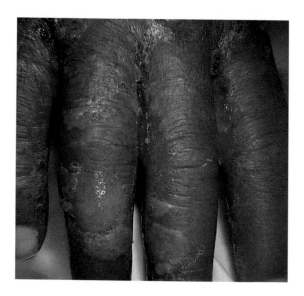

Figure 6.45
Unusual case of cryoglobulinemia

The punched-out ulcers in this 74-year-old woman suggested a number of possibilities, including vasculitis, infection, and factitial disease. Because of the sudden onset of her ulcers, she was admitted to the hospital. Work-up showed that she had cryoglobulinemia. She died shortly thereafter because of numerous medical problems.

Figure 6.46
Toxic epidermal necrolysis

After being given penicillin for a systemic infection, this patient developed generalized erythema followed by sloughing of the skin. The photograph shows areas denuded of skin. Biopsy was consistent with toxic epidermal necrolysis. This is a life-threatening condition with a mortality of more than 30%. Patients require very meticulous medical care and fluid replacement. Wound care is also important in these patients. Non-stick sheets and bandages are essential. Recent evidence supports the use of intravenous gamma globulin.

7 Neoplasms and ulcers

Introduction

Skin cancers are the most common form of malignancy, and metastasis to the skin, such as from lung, breast, lymphomas and leukemias (particularly myelomonocytic), is not uncommon. Certain conditions have to be present, however, for the development of ulcerations in the setting of malignancies in the skin. For the most part, this has to do with the size of the tumor or whether the cancer arises within pre-existing ulcerations. Neoplasms are highly dependent on angiogenesis and blood supply for continued and stable growth. Generally, it is when growth exceeds vascular supply that ulcers occur within neoplasms. In other situations, neoplasms develop within ulcers, such as the typical occurrence of squamous cell carcinoma in non-healing ulcers. A history of ionizing irradiation predisposes patients to the development of primary cutaneous malignancies at the site of radiation, even decades later.

The diagnosis of neoplasia in ulcers can be difficult, especially when the clinical picture is that of a leg ulcer. For example, basal cell carcinoma can present as granulation tissue-like material within venous ulcers, and is often associated with intermittent episodes of re-epithelialization. It is generally good practice to biopsy leg ulcers that have failed to heal. The timing of the biopsy is uncertain, however. Some clinicians suggest biopsying leg ulcers that have not shown evidence of healing for a period of 2–3 months. This is not unreasonable, but one must remain flexible about this. For example, a sampling problem exists; one biopsy does not necessarily exclude the presence of cancer. Moreover, as we have just stated, intermittent episodes of re-epithelialization can occur with malignant processes. Location of the ulceration is also important. Thus, an ulcerated lesion in areas other than the leg would immediately suggest the possibility of cancer, and a biopsy should be performed at the start of the evaluation. Another pitfall regarding biopsies of tumors is that a small punch biopsy of the edge of the wound can often be uninterpretable because of the associated inflammatory process and completely miss the tumor. If the clinical situation demands it (i.e. unclear diagnosis and failure to heal), one needs to perform an excisional biopsy that goes at least 1–2 cm beyond the wound's margins. Occasionally, the tumor is at the base of the wound. This situation arises in cases of recurrent cancers. Indeed, histologic findings of fibrosis or sclerosis can mislead the clinician into thinking that only a scar is present; the fibrosis may simply be a reaction to the tumor.

Ulcerated tumors can be very exudative and foul-smelling, features which can be a substantial management problem. This clinical picture is not uncommon with metastatic breast carcinomas and with certain lymphomas, such as cutaneous T-cell lymphomas. In end-stage cancer, and when the ulcerated lesions are extensive, the goal is to provide comfort to the patient and make wound management easier. Antiseptics, which are generally avoided for fear of inhibiting healing, can be helpful in this particular situation. Certain topical antibiotics, such as metronidazole, can also decrease the bacterial burden and improve the problem of odour control.

Clinical points

- Non-healing ulcers with exuberant granulation tissue should be biopsied to exclude basal cell carcinoma.
- Malignancies within ulcers arise more commonly when there has been prior ionizing radiation to the area.
- Intermittent re-epithelialization in non-healing wounds should raise the suspicion of an underlying malignancy.
- Cutaneous lymphomas are often purple in color and ulcerate as they enlarge.
- Unusual streaks of hyperpigmentation of the lower extremity may represent Kaposi's sarcoma.

- Kaposi's sarcoma is strongly associated with herpes virus type 8 infection.
- Squamous cell carcinomas can arise in chronic wounds and scars.
- Tumors infiltrating the skin can block lymphatic channels and cause a clinical picture of cutaneous edema.
- The diagnosis of lymphomas and other tumors within ulcers can be missed when the biopsy is small and only involves the inflammatory areas of the ulcer. When indicated, the biopsy should extend well beyond the ulcer's edge.
- Myelomonocytic leukemia commonly involves the skin.
- Ovarian tumors can metastasize to the umbilicus.

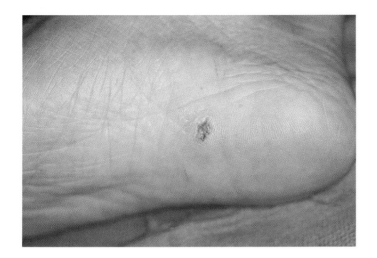

Figure 7.1
Adnexal tumor masquerading as an ulcer

This young man had a non-healing ulcer on his foot for about a year. The ulcer would occasionally re-epithelialize, only to break down again. When we saw him, we thought this ulcer could represent a non-melanotic melanoma or an appendegeal tumor. Indeed, a biopsy of the lesion seen in the photograph showed the typical histologic findings of syringocystadenoma papilliferum, which is a benign tumor, more commonly observed on the scalp. The lesion was completely excised. This case underscores the need for biopsy, especially when the location of the ulcer is atypical for common types of ulcerations, such as venous or diabetic etiology.

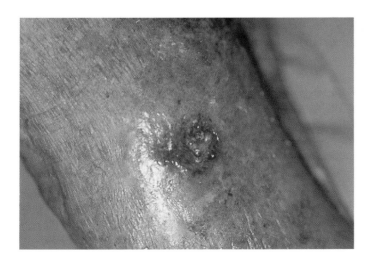

Figure 7.2a
Basal cell carcinoma

The next three photographs show non-healing ulcers of the leg complicated by the development of basal cell carcinomas. One should be alert to this possibility when, in addition to failure to heal, the ulcers show intermittent episodes of re-epithelialization, exuberant granulation tissue, or edges which appear to roll over onto the surrounding skin.

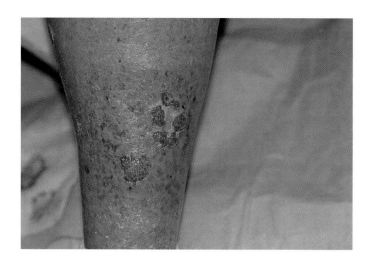

Figure 7.2b
Basal cell carcinoma

This patient was treated unsuccessfully with compression bandages, until it was recognized that the ulcers represented basal cell carcinomas. This complication is observed more commonly in patients who have received radiation to the leg or substantial solar damage.

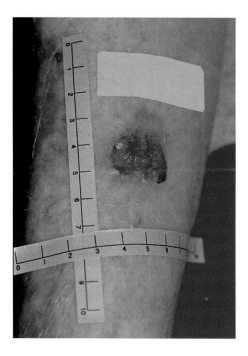

Figure 7.2c
Basal cell carcinoma

Exuberant granulation tissue with failure to re-epithelialize. Note that the edges of the wound appear to "invade" the surrounding skin. Biopsy showed basal cell carcinoma.

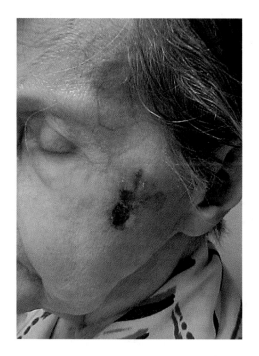

Figure 7.2d
Basal cell carcinoma

The patient had a "bump" on her cheek for at least 2 years. Over the last several months, it ulcerated. It was treated by excision and a cutaneous flap.

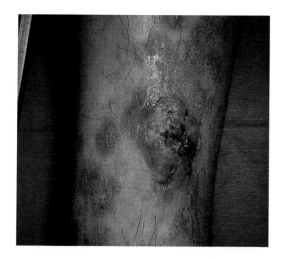

Figure 7.3
Squamous cell carcinoma

This elderly woman had numerous nodules and plaques on the leg. The ulcerated lesion was initially thought to represent a keratinous cyst. However, the histology showed that this was a squamous cell carcinoma. She had received radiation therapy to her leg decades earlier. The other nodules were also found to represent squamous cell carcinomas.

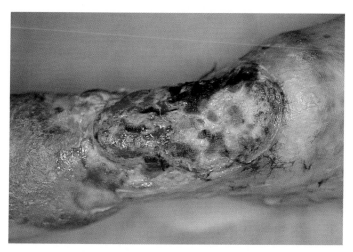

Figure 7.4a
Squamous cell carcinoma

This man had received a bayonet injury to both legs more than 20 years earlier. The wound never healed and he refused further treatment. Several years later, the wound began to enlarge and showed increasing amounts of exudate and necrosis. Multiple biopsies confirmed the clinical suspicion that this represented a squamous cell carcinoma.

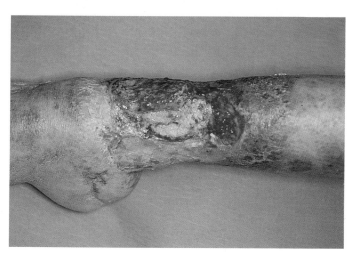

Figure 7.4b
Squamous cell carcinoma/Close-up

The patient vehemently refused amputation and was treated for a while with surgical debridement, occlusive dressings, and Mohs histographic surgery to decrease the tumor burden. However, the cancer extended to the bone and osteomyelitis was also present. He eventually agreed to bilateral amputation.

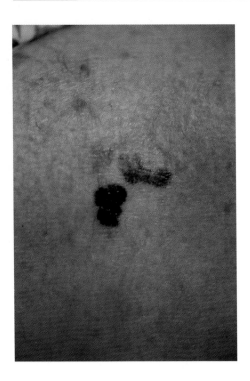

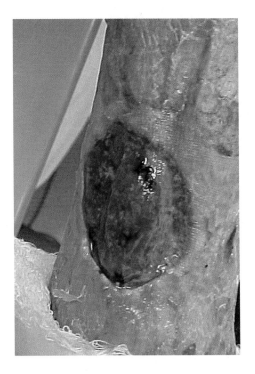

Figure 7.5a
Superficial spreading melanoma

Melanomas generally ulcerate only when
they get to a certain size and are nodular.
The lesions shown here are superficial
spreading melanomas. When excised at this
stage, there is still a good chance of cure.

Figure 7.5b
Metastatic melanoma to the skin

Melanomas commonly metastasize to the
brain, lung, and liver. In some unusual cases,
as in this 67-year-old woman, they may
metastasize to the skin alone. Over the last
few years since the initial diagnosis of
melanoma, she keeps getting recurrent and
deep tumors, which require extensive
excision down to muscle. Here one sees a
large excision on the lower part of her leg.
The underlying muscle is clearly visible. The
wound will require grafting.

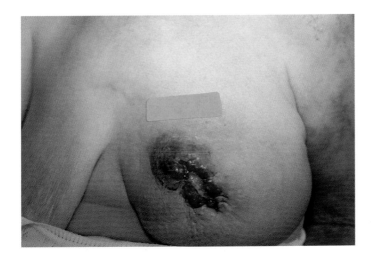

Figure 7.6
Breast carcinoma

The patient has breast carcinoma extending to the skin. The lesions are typically quite hard and may assume this purple appearance. Ulceration is a common complication when the tumor reaches a certain size. The tumor infiltrating the skin also blocks lymphatic channels, thus leading to substantial dermal and subcutaneous edema.

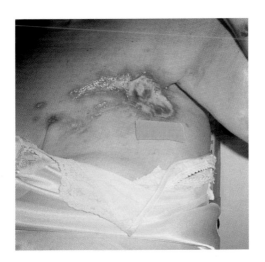

Figure 7.7
Breast carcinoma after mastectomy

Local recurrence of breast carcinoma after mastectomy. Although there is redness, there are no other signs of infection. These ulcerations can be quite exudating, however, and may require antibiotic treatment. On palpation, the lesion is quite hard and only moderately tender.

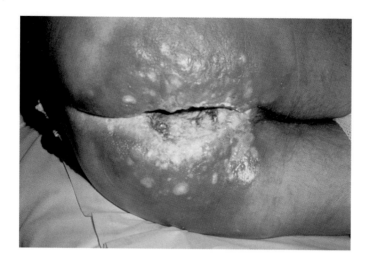

Figure 7.8
Rectal carcinoma

Local recurrence in the perianal area due to a rectal malignancy. The entire perineum is infiltrated by tumor cells and, not surprisingly, the area is quite tender. The region immediately adjacent to the anus is ulcerated and weeping. Approaches to help the patient's pain and situation might include gel dressing to the ulcerated area, strong systemic narcotics, and a pressure-relieving surface.

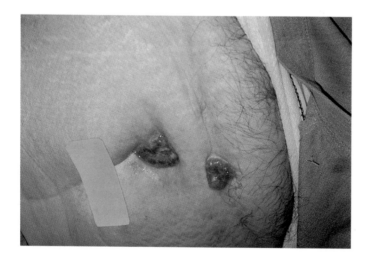

Figure 7.9
Ovarian cancer

This patient had advanced ovarian cancer. The purple, ulcerated nodules seen in the photograph represent extension of the tumor to the abdominal wall and skin. Involvement of the skin within the umbilicus is a well-described clinical feature of metastatic ovarian cancer.

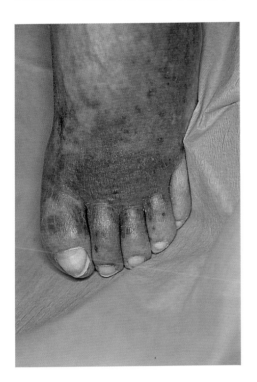

Figure 7.10
Kaposi's sarcoma

These purple nodules on the foot are quite typical of Kaposi's sarcoma. In this case, the patient was of Mediterranean ethnic origin, and thus more likely to develop this tumor. He did not have evidence of infection with the human immunodeficiency virus. It is now known that Kaposi's sarcoma is probably the result of infection with herpes virus type 8. In some cases the hyperpigmentation associated with this tumor may be confused with that observed with venous insufficiency. Occasionally, one has to biopsy the involved skin to make this differentiation.

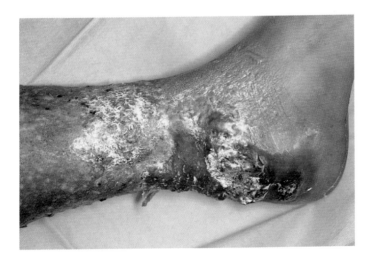

Figure 7.11a
Kaposi's sarcoma and AIDS

This 29-year-old man with AIDS presented with these ulcerations on the lower leg and with very hard skin involving most of the leg. Biopsy showed Kaposi's sarcoma.

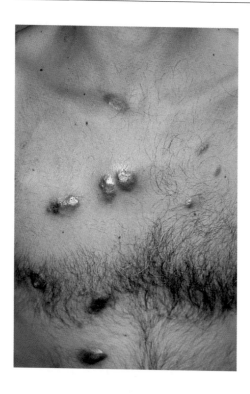

Figure 7.11b
Kaposi's sarcoma and AIDS/Chest involvement

The patient also had large nodules on his chest. Some of them were linear in shape, which is rather characteristic of Kaposi's sarcoma occurring in AIDS patients.

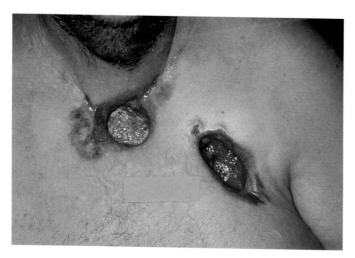

Figure 7.12
Non-Hodgkin's lymphoma

These large tumors ulcerated and developed sinus tracts between them. As with other lymphomas, the purple color of the lesions is very helpful in pointing to the diagnosis.

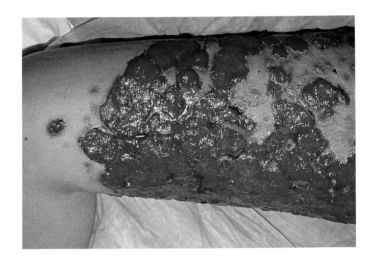

Figure 7.13
Large cell lymphoma in a child

This child was found to have a CD30- and CD4-positive lymphoma involving the entire thigh and lower abdomen. The tumors have ulcerated and have become a difficult management problem because of the bloody exudate. Foam dressings and compression bandages can be used here to help absorb exudate and protect the area from trauma.

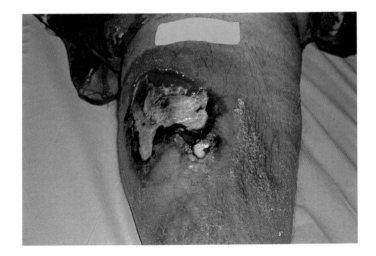

Figure 7.14
Multiple myeloma

This necrobiotic xanthogranuloma was present in a patient with multiple myeloma. These rare tumors can appear as isolated, as in this case, or multiple lesions. No satisfactory treatment is available. In this case, she was thought to have an infection at first, until a biopsy was obtained.

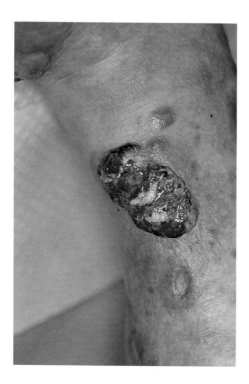

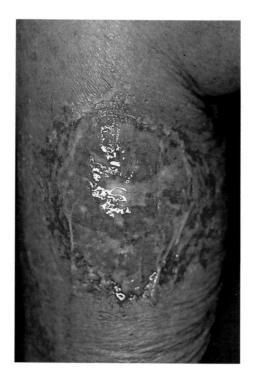

Figure 7.15
Cutaneous T-cell lymphoma and tumors

The cutaneous tumors in this adult were
mostly on the back of his right leg. In spite
of the presence of this cancer, one can see
strips of epithelium running across the
wound. This is also commonly observed in
ulcers containing basal cell carcinomas.
Therefore, partial and intermittent re-
epithelialization should not fool one into
thinking that cancer is not present.

Figure 7.16
Cutaneous T-cell lymphoma

This painful tumor on the lower leg
developed rapidly (within weeks) in this
patient with pre-existing cutaneous T-cell
lymphoma. Bacterial contamination was
managed with the topical use of silver
sulfadiazine. Once the infection or wound
contamination is gone, one can manage these
lesions with occlusive dressings, such as
films. She was eventually treated with
electron beam therapy, which healed this
ulcerated tumor.

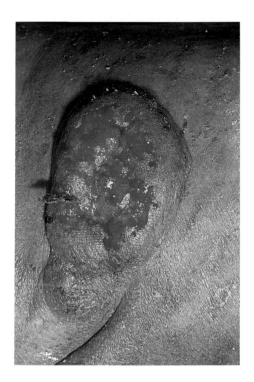

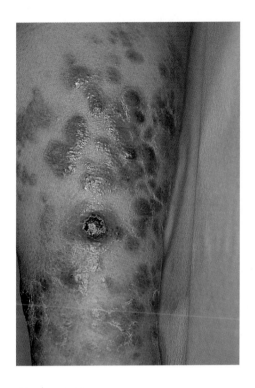

Figure 7.17
Cutaneous T-cell lymphoma and ulceration

The patient was 68 years old and had cutaneous T-cell lymphoma diagnosed 30 years earlier. Over the last few years, she began to have cutaneous tumors. This particular one has ulcerated. It was treated with radiation therapy.

Figure 7.18a
B-cell lymphoma

This 80-year-old man from South America was thought to have Kaposi's sarcoma or pseudoangiosarcoma. He had radiation and systemic chemotherapy. Upon our evaluation, he was initially thought to have tumor stage cutaneous T-cell lymphoma, based only on the histology and immunohistochemistry. Further studies, however, including gene rearrangements, showed that this was a B-cell lymphoma.

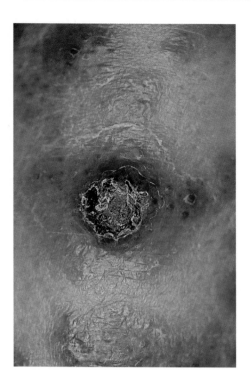

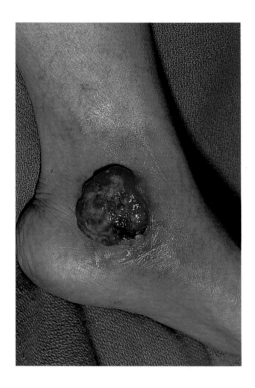

Figure 7.18b
B-cell lymphoma/Close-up

The close-up here shows the scaling that occasionally surrounds rapidly growing tumors or lesions with substantial lymphocytic infiltration. This case also highlights the difficulties in arriving at the correct diagnosis in some patients with lymphomas. This patient was eventually treated with electron beam therapy. Topical treatment with nitrogen mustard and systemic therapy with retinoids did not help.

Figure 7.19
B-cell lymphoma resembling granulation tissue

This middle-aged woman had an ulcer on the medial aspect of the leg that was initially thought to represent exuberant granulation tissue. Biopsy and molecular studies showed that it was a B-cell lymphoma.

8 Practical points

Introduction

The title of this section does not imply that the previous ones were not "practical" and merely theoretical in content. Nevertheless, there are some aspects of wound management that are essential elements of wound care and are common to many different types of ulcers. Hence, these "points" are described in this section.

There are extensive reviews and guides on the subject of wound dressings, but it may be useful to provide a brief summary here. The clinical photographs in this section will give some clues and advice on their use. There are now hundreds of different brands of wound dressings. Learning about these dressings may at first seem a daunting task. However, based on composition, transparency, and adherence properties, there are only a finite number of dressing categories from which to choose. In this section, we describe the use of transparent films, foams, hydrogels, hydrocolloids, and alginates. Some dressings are created by combinations. For example, an island dressing has a central absorbent portion surrounded by an adhesive component.

Films are generally composed of polyurethane and are adhesive and transparent. They are ideal for erosions or shallow ulcers and are not able to absorb exudate. They are usually used as a primary dressing (i.e. directly in contact with the wound). However, they can also be used as a secondary dressing to keep other dressings in place. Foam dressings are also generally composed of polyurethane. Unlike films, they are mostly non-adhesive and are not transparent. They can absorb substantial amounts of exudate and thus can be used for deeper and moderately exudative wounds. Hydrocolloids are a third major category of wound dressings. They are composed, for the most part, of carboxymethyl cellulose. They adhere to the skin surrounding the wound and "melt" into the wound. In addition to having some absorptive properties, they seem to be particularly useful in causing painless debridement. Hydrogels are made of polyethylene and up to 90% water. Most products in this category are not adhesive but some new products have an adhesive border. We have used hydrogels very successfully in the management of painful ulcers and in the treatment of ulcers surrounded by substantial dermatitis. It should also be noted that hydrogels, besides being available as a sheet (the traditional form), are also available in an amorphous form. Hydrogels, because of their high water content, can actually hydrate wounds. In doing so, however, they can cause some maceration of the surrounding tissues. Alginate dressings are derived from seaweed. They are ideal for highly exudative wounds. It should be kept in mind that the field of wound dressings evolves very quickly. For example, in the last few years, new categories of dressings have emerged, such as collagens, hydrofibers, superabsorbents, and hydropolymers.

There is more to wound care than just dressings, however. Wound care has to do with providing the ideal microenvironment to the wound, optimizing wound closure, and addressing the needs of the patient. All of these aspects have to be taken into account. Thus, in two patients with identical wounds, management may be different because of the clinical and patient-specific circumstances. We hope that this section will highlight some of these points and provide a useful perspective.

Clinical points

- It is wise to have a wide variety of dressing types available and be willing to experiment to find the best one for each individual clinical situation.
- Keeping close at hand a list showing the different types of dressings available and their properties is useful.
- The package insert for each new dressing must be read carefully. Some dressings have one side that is absorbent and one side (away from the wound) which is not water-permeable.
- When applying a hydrogel sheet dressing, one must be careful to remove the thin film from the side that will be in contact with the wound. The outer film can be left on to keep the dressing moist.
- For a heavily exudating wound with an offensive odor, a foam dressing with an activated carbon layer is useful for absorbing organic odors. An alternative approach is to use topical metronidazole.
- Hydrogen peroxide can be used to break down the absorbent component of certain polyurethane dressings when these need to be removed.
- Patients need to be informed about the possible odor and the rather extensive and pus-like wound fluid which accumulates under hydrocolloid dressings.
- Although each type of occlusive dressing comes with certain recommendations concerning how long it can stay on the wound, in general it is best not to remove the dressing until leakage of the wound fluid occurs. Premature removal of the dressing leads to disruption of re-epithelializing tissue.
- Compression bandages should be applied from the toes to below the knee and fully enclose the heel. "Heel sparing", however, can be useful in patients with combined venous and arterial disease.
- Rigid compression bandages (e.g. Unna boot) are probably not effective in non-ambulatory patients. In these patients, elastic bandages are preferred.
- It is wise to be as specific as possible when instructing patients about leg elevation for venous insufficiency. The expression "toes above nose" seems to deliver the message in a more explicit way.
- A stocking butler should be kept in the office in order to demonstrate how useful it can be in applying stockings.
- In order to facilitate compliance with dressings and bandages, it is best to give patients a hand-out listing the addresses of several local pharmacies or suppliers which carry the harder-to-find items.
- Hydrocolloid dressings are best for painless wound debridement, while calcium alginate dressings and foams are good for highly exudative wounds.
- Adhesive dressings should be used with caution in patients (especially the elderly) with very fragile skin.
- Cadexomer iodine is an ideal agent for exudative and contaminated wounds. It is best to change the dressing daily, both for effectiveness and because dried cadexomer iodine is more difficult to remove.
- Multilayered bandages are ideal in patients whose legs have an "inverted bowling pin" appearance and where other types of bandages tend to slip down.

- One simple way to avoid injury to the leg when removing a leg bandage is to pull the outer wrap away from the leg while cutting it.
- Ulcer pain can often be managed with the use of occlusive dressings alone.
- An effective way to minimize pain during debridement is to apply EMLA cream to the ulcer for 30–45 min before the procedure.
- Film dressings are ideal for controlling the intense pain of fissures of the hands, as in patients with severe dermatitis or psoriasis.
- Dermatitis of the leg is often best controlled by the use of hydrogels.

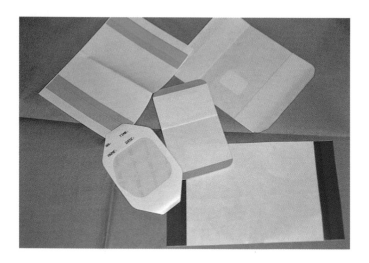

Figure 8.1
Film dressings

These polyurethane dressings are generally transparent and adhere to the skin surrounding the ulceration. They are very good for shallow wounds with little exudate. Only a handful are shown in this photograph, and each brand will have its own specific advantages or special indications.

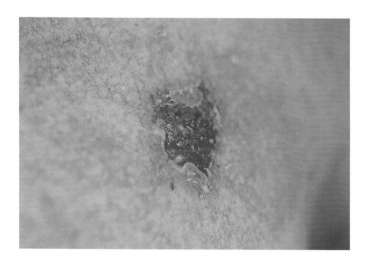

Figure 8.2
Erosion

This wound is caused by pemphigus vulgaris. It is a superficial erosion and needs to be protected and kept in a moist environment for optimal wound healing. One of the film dressings shown above is ideal for these wounds.

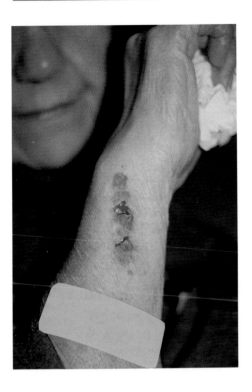

Figure 8.3
Erosion of fragile skin

The skin in the elderly or in patients on corticosteroids (including inhaled preparations for asthma) is very fragile and tears easily. Adherent film dressings are ideal for these wounds but they should be kept on until healing has occurred. Premature removal can lead to further damage to the skin.

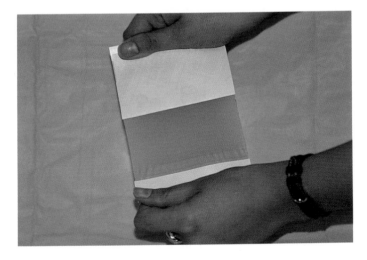

Figure 8.4
Film application

When applying a film dressing, the backing is removed and the adherent side is placed against the wound. One must be careful so that the adherent portions of the dressing do not stick to each other. In this particular film, the green portion is not adherent and can be used to handle the dressing during application.

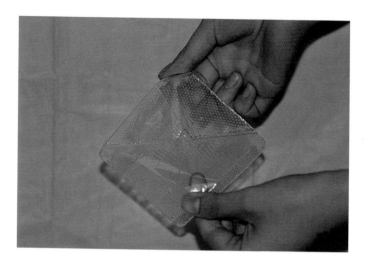

Figure 8.5
Gel dressing

These non-adherent semi-transparent dressings are made of polyethylene and consist of large amounts of water. They require irradiation for sterilization. On either side of the dressing is a polyurethane film. Generally, one removes the film side that will be in contact with the wound. By keeping the upper film on the dressing, one avoids excessive drying of the polyethylene portion. These gels absorb considerable amounts of exudate and can be used in some exudative wounds. In our experience, they are also excellent for the treatment of dermatitis. Hydrogels provide a soothing relief from pain, and can be kept refrigerated to give a cooling effect when applied to the skin.

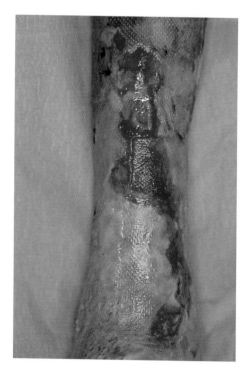

Figure 8.6
Painful venous ulcer

Although this ulcer is healing, there is a considerable amount of pain. A hydrogel dressing is a good way to deal with it. Some areas, especially superiorly, show a yellow and necrotic wound base, and the dressing should also be able to provide autolytic debridement. Because of the pain, one should keep in mind the possibility of infection; sometimes, pain is the only clue to this, especially in the elderly.

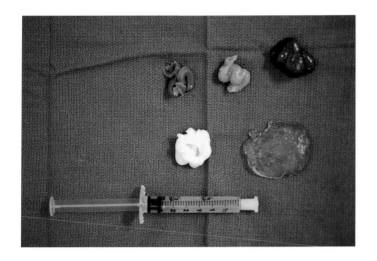

Figure 8.7a
Absorptive wound dressings/Other gels

This photograph shows several types of gel materials that can be used to fill the wound, provide an absorptive function and, in some cases, debridement and wound stimulatory effects.

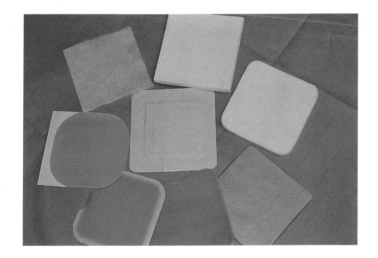

Figure 8.7b
Absorptive wound dressings

There are other additional types of dressings that are able to handle considerable amounts of exudate. The photograph shows a small sample of hydrocolloids (top four), foams (one in the center and two at left bottom) and calcium alginate (right bottom). There are many variations of these dressings. They are very useful in effecting pain relief, autolytic debridement, and stimulation of granulation tissue.

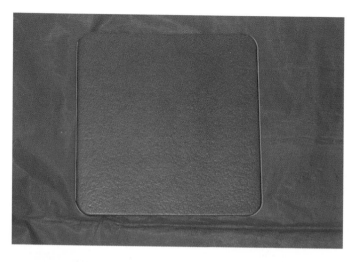

Figure 8.8a
Hydrocolloid dressing

This is a typical hydrocolloid. The underside backing is removed and that side is applied to the wound. Like many other hydrocolloids, it is adhesive and absorbs exudate. When first applied, it may not adhere well until it is heated by body temperature or the hand of the person applying it.

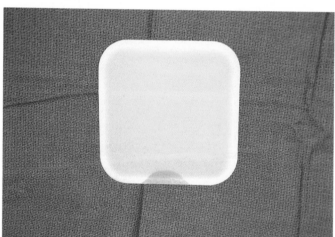

Figure 8.8b
Another hydrocolloid

There are many different versions of hydrocolloids. The tapered edges of this particular one help in the application and in keeping it adherent to the skin around the wound.

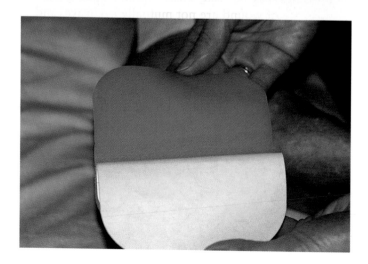

Figure 8.8c
Hydrocolloid dressing/Application

This photograph shows how the actual hydrocolloid dressing (top) is removed from its white backing (bottom), which is discarded.

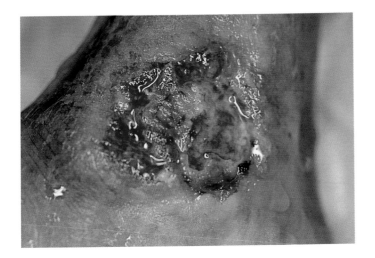

Figure 8.9
Necrotic purulent wound

This is the type of wound that can benefit from the use of a hydrocolloid. The dressing will typically remove the necrotic tissue and build up a good granulating base. The wound is not infected, but its surface is colonized with bacteria. Many clinicians are still afraid of applying a dressing that makes this wound moist, for they fear that infection will occur. However, vast clinical experience shows that it is safe and beneficial to occlude such wounds.

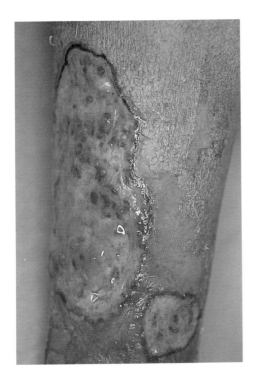

Figure 8.10
Heavily exudative and colonized wound

There could be considerable controversy as to how this wound should be handled. The wound is very painful and it may well be necessary to debride it surgically. Another way would be to apply cadexomer iodine dressings, which are antimicrobial and absorb exudate. Some clinicians would use occlusive dressings, such as a hydrocolloid. Foam dressings may be used. These ways of dealing with this type of wound are not mutually exclusive, and often a sequence of dressings is required during treatment. Whirlpool treatment is also a useful option.

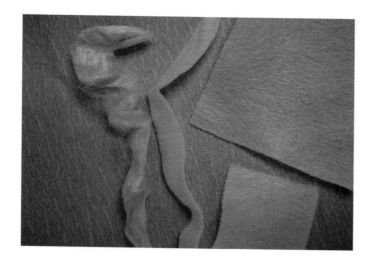

Figure 8.11
Calcium alginate

These dressings are extremely useful for highly exudative wounds. As shown here, there are several different types to fit the clinical needs, i.e. sheets and ropes for large wounds, draining sinuses, etc. The calcium in the dressing is exchanged for sodium, which is present in the wound exudate. For this reason, calcium alginate dressings should not be used in non-exudative wounds.

Figure 8.12
Foam dressing

These polyurethane materials are also very helpful for exudative wounds. They have the advantage of not adhering to the wound or surrounding skin, which makes them attractive when dealing with fragile skin in the elderly or with wounds that are re-epithelializing very slowly.

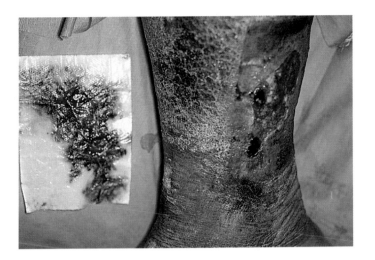

Figure 8.13
Wound exudate

This is the appearance of wound exudate in a colonized venous ulcer. In this case, the dressing was a non-adherent pad with little if any capacity to absorb exudate. A hydrocolloid or foam would have been very useful in this situation and would have probably stimulated the formation of granulation tissue.

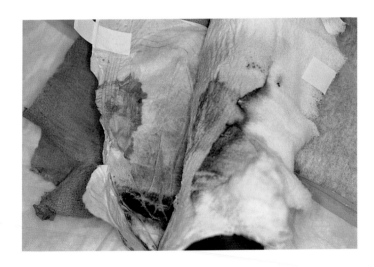

Figure 8.14
Soiled dressings

The photograph shows the appearance of a compression bandage that is being cut and removed. As shown, there can be considerable exudate that accumulates within the bandages. The drainage is often foul-smelling, which can be very upsetting to patients and can fool inexperienced clinicians into thinking that the wound is infected. A way to deal with this problem is to use an absorbent wound dressing, such as foams, hydrocolloids, alginates. Other clinicians have used antimicrobial agents or absorbant material within the bandages to decrease the number of bacteria and the foul odor.

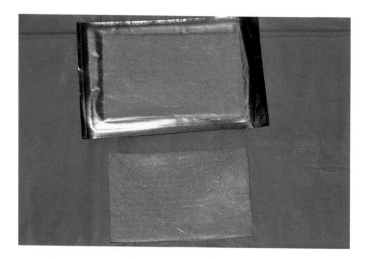

Figure 8.15a
Collagen–alginate dressing

Other types of dressings and combinations, both in structure and function, are also becoming popular. This particular one combines collagen and a calcium alginate material. It has the potential to absorb considerable amounts of exudate while also providing new matrix material to the wound.

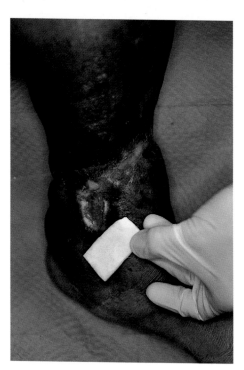

Figure 8.15b
Collagen–alginate dressing/Granulating venous ulcer

The collagen–alginate combination is being used in this difficult-to-heal wound that has been present for many months.

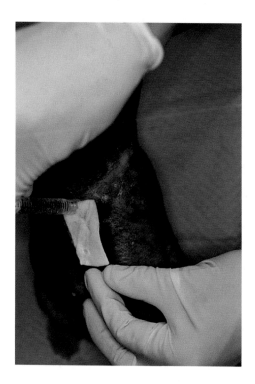

Figure 8.15c
Collagen–alginate dressing/Application

After the wound becomes less exudative, it is generally necessary to use a saline solution when applying an alginate-containing dressing.

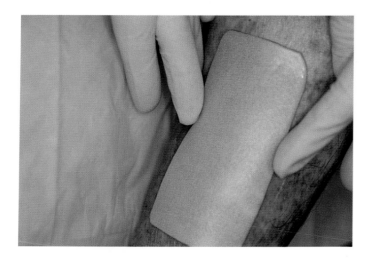

Figure 8.16
Hydrocolloid in place

As mentioned earlier, it is a good idea to hold down all sides of the dressing and round the corners when applying a hydrocolloid dressing. This approach of slightly warming the material helps secure it in place.

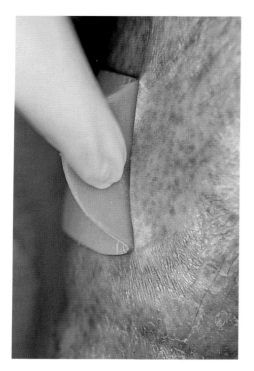

Figure 8.17a
Removal of hydrocolloid

To remove a hydrocolloid dressing, one can can roll it off gently and slowly so as not to pull off any new epithelial tissue. Sometimes, clinicians apply warm saline to it or even inject it into the dressing. However, the key issue is not to remove the dressing unless it needs to be removed; removal is safer when there is leakage of exudate or when the part directly over the ulcer bubbles up because of the accumulation of exudate.

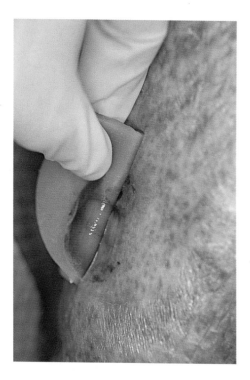

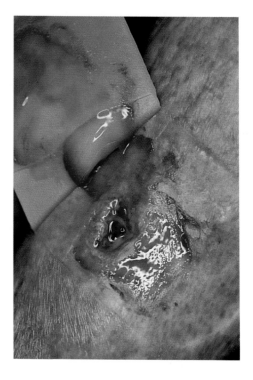

Figure 8.17b
Removal of hydrocolloid/Exudate

Here one can see that the area over the wound contains wound fluid and is no longer adherent. This fluid is a mixture of wound fluid as well as part of the hydrocolloid material.

Figure 8.17c
Removal of hydrocolloid/Exudate

When using this and other types of occlusive dressings, it is important to warn the patient that fluid (both from the wound and the dressing material) will accumulate and actually become quite malodorous. Failure to warn patients will probably lead them to believe that the wound has become infected. This is not the case. Also, there is an exudative phase that starts after the first application of occlusive dressing and which can last several weeks.

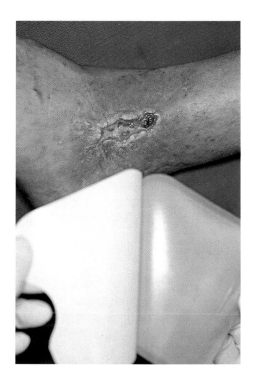

Figure 8.18a
Use of hydrocolloid/Application

The white backing of the dressing is removed and discarded and the tacky (adherent) side of the hydrocolloid is applied to the wound.

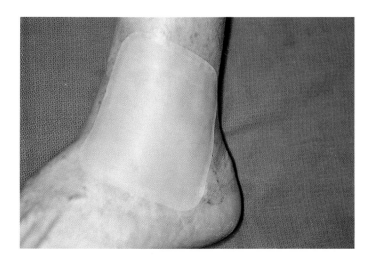

Figure 8.18b
Use of hydrocolloid/Dressing in place

There should be a generous border of the dressing around the wound to get the dressing to adhere well and also to contain the exudate.

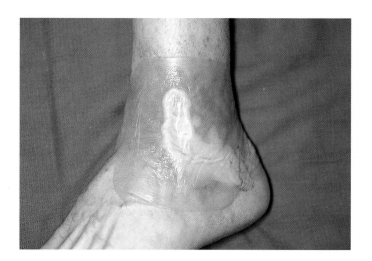

Figure 8.18c
Use of hydrocolloid/After 3 days

It is a good idea to have the largest border at the dependent edge where drainage is most likely to run out.

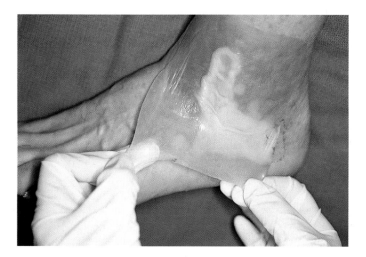

Figure 8.18d
Use of hydrocolloid/Removal

The dressing should be removed when drainage begins to leak out from the edge of the dressing. To minimize the force exerted on the surrounding skin, the recommendation is to lift the dressing and remove it by holding the free edge close to the skin.

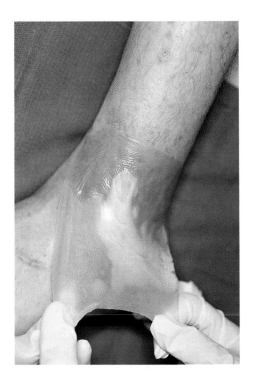

Figure 8.18e
Use of hydrocolloid/Removal

This shows the next stage of removal as the dressing is lifted by maintaining the free edge close to the skin.

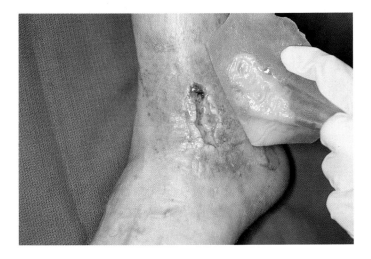

Figure 8.18f
Use of hydrocolloid/Removal

The dressing is almost completely removed. When the ulcer is first exposed, there can be considerable foul odor; it is best to warn patients about this.

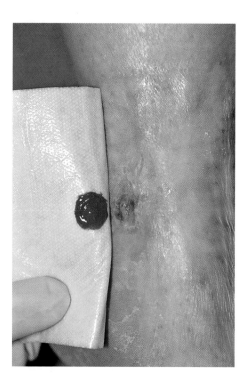

Figure 8.19a
Cadexomer iodine/Application

There are other ways to debride wounds and stimulate granulation tissue, besides the use of occlusive dressings. Here we have used cadexomer iodine. This preparation consists of 0.9% iodine incorporated into cadexomer beads. When this agent is applied to an exudative wound, the iodine is slowly exchanged for wound fluid and released into the wound. Cadexomer iodine gel is usually applied by spreading a thin layer of it on a non-adherent dressing. Only enough cadexomer iodine to cover the wound should be used.

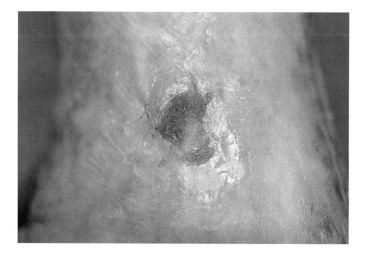

Figure 8.19b
Cadexomer iodine/After several days

The iodine is slowly released into the exudative wound and the gel becomes a light color, as shown here. This is a signal for removal of the material and, if needed, a new application. From a practical standpoint, it is probably easier to instruct the patient or the visiting nurse to remove cadexomer iodine and reapply it daily, rather than waiting for this change in color. Also, we have found that dried cadexomer iodine is more difficult to remove.

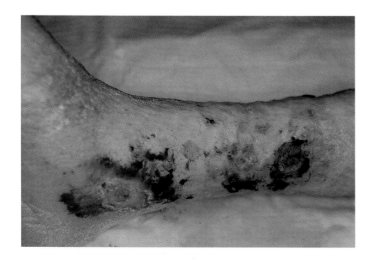

Figure 8.20a
Cadexomer iodine removal

This is an example where cadexomer iodine was applied improperly by including the surrounding skin. What happens is that the material hardens on non-ulcerated skin and becomes difficult to remove.

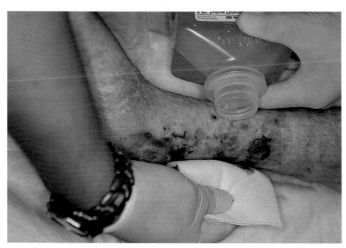

Figure 8.20b
Cadexomer iodine removal/Saline irrigation

Soaking the material with saline tends to make removal of the gel easier.

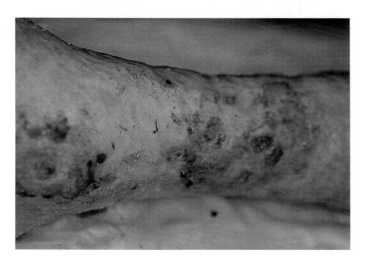

Figure 8.20c
Cadexomer iodine removal/After saline irrigation

There is still residual cadexomer iodine material which is now stuck to the scaling skin. It is best to leave this alone, or else one might cause damage to the skin. The wound bed looks very good and, in fact, there is new epithelium covering these wounds.

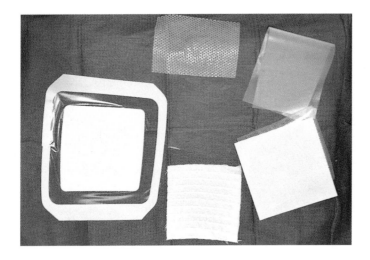

Figure 8.21
Other dressings

There is a wide variety of wound dressings, with different structure and function capabilities. This photograph shows a few of them which can be used for different purposes. For example, the island dressing on the left can achieve moist wound healing as well as control the exudate. Others shown here can be used for donor sites and for painful shallow wounds. The point should be made that the process of wound healing is really a spectrum, thus often requiring different types of dressings at different stages.

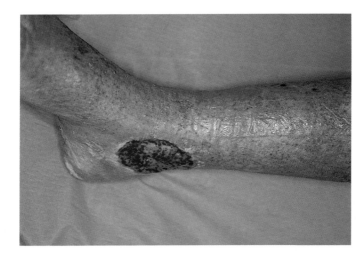

Figure 8.22a
Compression treatment

Compression is the standard treatment for venous ulcers. The ulcer shown in this photograph is being treated with a zinc oxide-impregnated bandage (Unna boot). Ulcers near or below the malleolus are difficult to heal, perhaps because compression is less reliable in this location. This patient is responding favorably to compression, and the ulcer bed shows granulation tissue. However, the edges of the wound are rather steep and do not yet exhibit that flattening associated with the process of re-epithelialization.

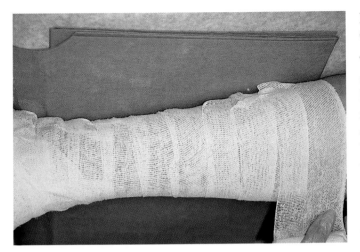

Figure 8.22b
Compression treatment/Unna boot

This bandage is generally applied with a 50% spiral overlap, although we have recently started to apply it in a figure of eight, which allows a more even distribution of the bandage. The Unna boot is an inelastic bandage that works best in ambulatory patients, because its mechanism of action has to do with pressing of the leg against the semi-rigid structure of the bandage. The Unna boot, with or without an additional elastic bandage, is favored in the USA, while many European clinicians prefer elastic compression bandages. However, there are no reliable data to show that one method of compression (elastic versus inelastic) is more effective than the other

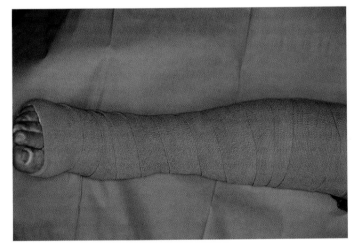

Figure 8.22c
Compression treatment/Unna boot

In the last several years, clinicians have combined the use of an Unna boot with an overlying elastic bandage, as shown in this photograph. Compression bandages are traditionally applied from the toes, including the heel, to just below the knee. Interestingly, some clinicians have recently suggested that exclusion of the heel from bandaging may be advantageous; presumably, this allows safer use of compression in patients with concomitant arterial disease and may improve ankle motion and calf muscle pump action. It is also good to keep in mind that there are studies suggesting that moist wound dressings should remain a part of wound care for venous ulcers being treated with compression bandages.

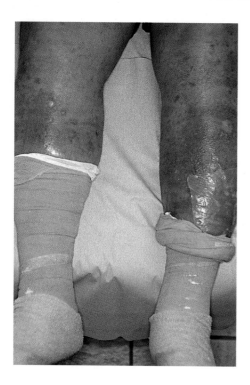

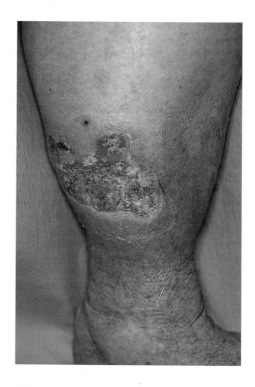

Figure 8.23
Compression/Inadequate results

This Unna boot did not stay in place due to several reasons. The patient has severe edema and probably needed to have the bandage changed more frequently than weekly. What happens is that compression reduces edema and the rigid bandage becomes loose. Also, it seems that the bandage was not applied all the way to the knee; anchoring the bandage above the calf muscles keeps it from slipping down. An additional reason for failure of the Unna boot or other similar bandages to stay on is the actual shape of the leg in some patients with venous disease.

Figure 8.24
Unusually shaped leg

On legs with small ankle circumference and very large calves ("champagne-bottle" or "inverted bowling pin" shaped legs), it is difficult to get an Unna boot to stay in place and also difficult to get the appropriate distribution of compression. This patient requires a different method of applying compression, one which takes into account this abnormal leg shape. Multi-layered elastic bandages would be more beneficial, because one of the layers is meant to "fill in" the concave areas of the leg and compensate for the abnormal leg shape.

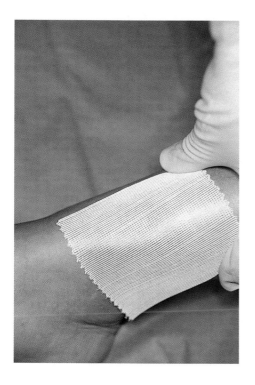

Figure 8.25a
Four-layer bandaging/Primary dressing

The primary dressing is applied over the wound. A number of dressings can be used for this purpose and their choice is dictated by the characteristics of the wound (i.e. exudative, need for debridement, etc.)

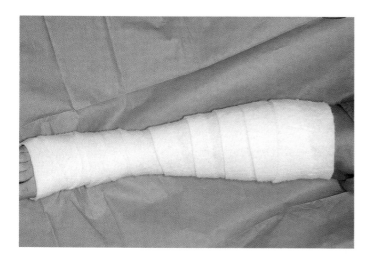

Figure 8.25b
Four-layer bandaging/First layer

The first layer, made of cotton-type material (as under casts), protects the leg and can be applied to make the shape of the leg more evenly tubular, thus preparing for proper compression.

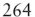

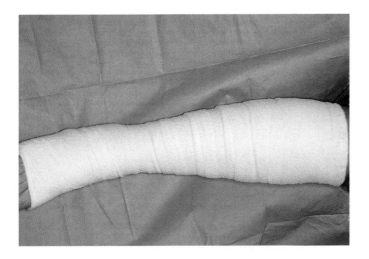

Figure 8.25c
Four-layer bandaging/Second layer

This can be applied without compression (there are different modifications of these systems) and helps keep the previous bandage in place and smooth it out.

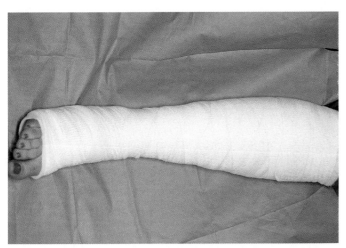

Figure 8.25d
Four-layer bandaging/Third layer

This particular elastic layer is applied in a figure of eight, which helps it from slipping and ensures adequate compression.

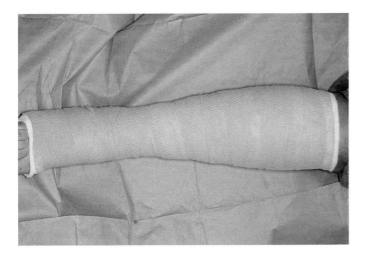

Figure 8.25e
Four-layer bandaging/Fourth layer

The final elastic compression bandage is applied at a 50% overlap and tension. Some of these bandages are self-adherent, while others require tape to secure them in place.

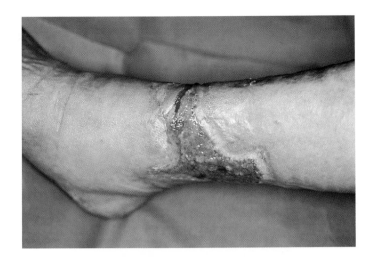

Figure 8.26a
Scissor injury

This occurred while removing an Unna boot with scissors that did not have a blunt leading edge.

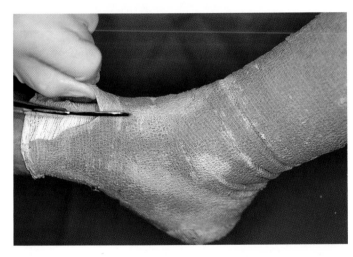

Figure 8.26b
Avoiding scissor injury

One simple way to avoid injury to the leg when removing a leg bandage is to pull the outer wrap away from the leg while cutting it.

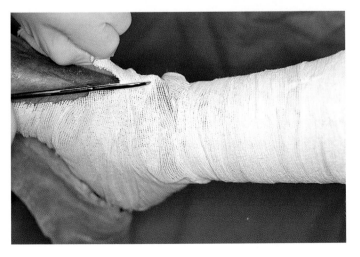

Figure 8.26c
Avoiding scissor injury/Further removal

The same procedure is used with the inner wrap, pulling it away from the leg and cutting with blunt-nosed, sharp-edged bandage scissors. We recommend using the thumb to get under the dressing and to pull it away from the skin. We also recommend asking the patient where the wound is, in case one is not familiar with the patient. One can then choose to cut the bandages in a path that avoids the wound.

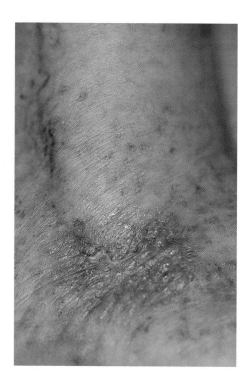

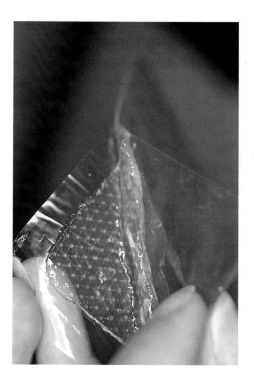

Figure 8.27a
Shallow but painful

It is easy to minimize the clinical significance
of the shallow wound seen in this
photograph. However, such small wounds
surrounded by small areas of pigmentation,
probably representing previous injury from
lividoid vasculitis, are very painful. Occlusive
dressings can help the pain.

Figure 8.27b
Shallow but painful/Hydrogel treatment

When applying a hydrogel sheet dressing,
one must remember to remove the membrane
from the side that will be applied next to the
patient's wound. Leaving the other side
intact will prevent the hydrogel from drying
out.

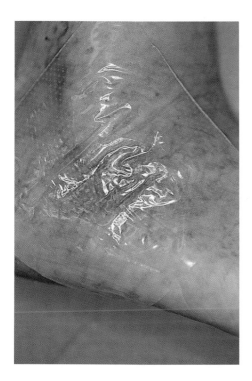

Figure 8.27c
Shallow but painful/Hydrogel applied

These dressings are very soothing when used on a painful ulcer. They can also be cooled before application, which provides added cooling relief.

Figure 8.28a
Radiation injury

This man had a liver transplant and required multiple fluoroscopic examinations. Although this is not commonly known, exposure to such examinations can cause radiation injury. This painful wound developed in the midst of the area affected by the radiation. The tissue around the wound is fibrotic and shows telengiectasia. The ulcer itself has a poor bed, even after several attempts at surgical debridement.

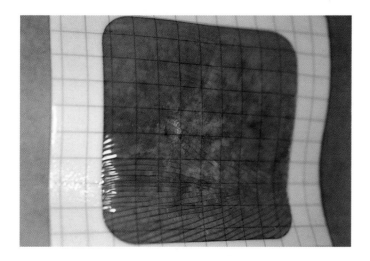

Figure 8.28b
Radiation injury/Dressing application

There were two problems in choosing a dressing for this wound. One is that the wound was on the back, so a non-adherent dressing would have to be taped in place. The second problem was that tape or strongly adherent dressings could damage the surrounding skin even further. In this case, an island hydrogel was used because it has an adherent border which allows easier removal. At the same time, the hydrogel provides pain relief. It is transparent, thus allowing wound inspection without removal. Moreover, the grid on the dressing can be useful in wound measurement.

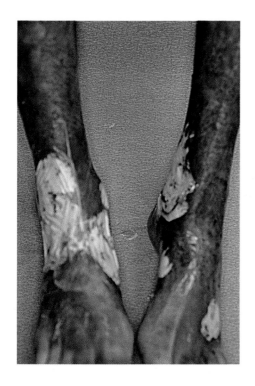

Figure 8.29
Chemical injury

The patient developed extremely painful ulcers after exposure to a chemical from a fire extinguisher. Several grafting procedures have not succeeded in healing or maintaining the ulcer healed. Similarly, a multitude of dressings had been tried, but his pain remained intolerable. EMLA cream, which contains three different anesthetic agents, was applied nightly and helped relieve his pain. The picture shows the cream in place. Dressings are then applied on top of the cream. Thus far, we have not seen hypersensitivity problems or serious untoward reactions with the use of this agent. Rarely, patients have complained of burning and have had to stop the use of EMLA.

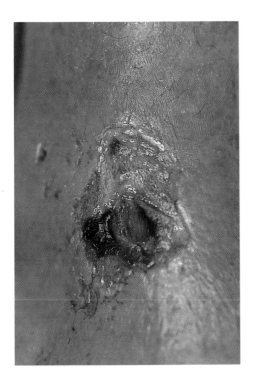

Figure 8.30a
Debridement

This man has necrotic and painful ulcers which are most likely due to cryofibrinogenemia. The ulcer requires debridement. The histology of a biopsy from the wound edge showed dermal thrombi.

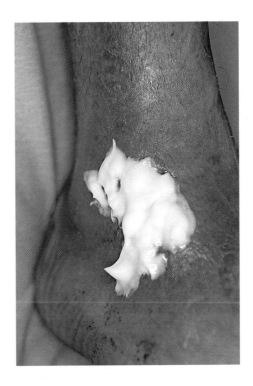

Figure 8.30b
Debridement/Managing pain

An effective way to minimize the pain caused by debridement is to apply EMLA cream to the ulcer for 30–45 min prior to the treatment.

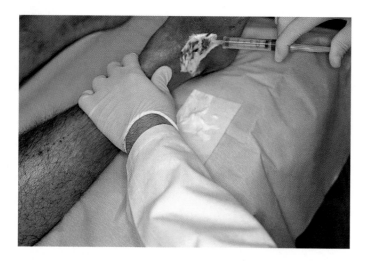

Figure 8.30c
Debridement/Managing pain

The EMLA cream often provides sufficient anesthesia for debridement. If more extensive debridement is necessary, the injection of an anesthetic agent will be less painful once the area has been primed with the EMLA cream.

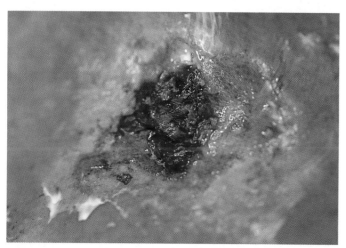

Figure 8.30d
Debridement/Managing pain

This is the appearance of the wound after debridement. The dark eschar and the necrotic tissue have been removed. Although occlusive dressings can also be used to cause painless debridement, they work rather slowly.

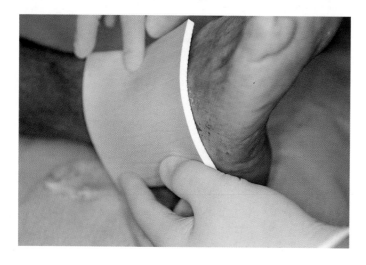

Figure 8.30e
Debridement/Managing pain

A foam dressing can be used after debridement to absorb the drainage, relieve pain, and provide an environment conducive to healing.

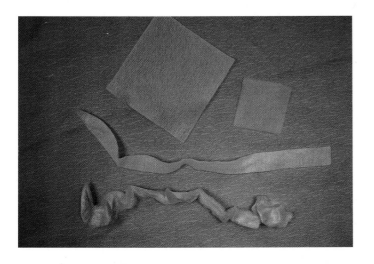

Figure 8.31
Calcium alginate dressings

Such material comes in several forms, different sizes of sheets as well as rope forms that one can easily pack into a wound. Calcium alginate can absorb a great deal of exudate.

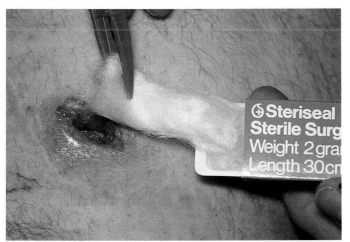

Figure 8.32
Calcium alginate packing

The material is being inserted in a wound sinus to absorb drainage.

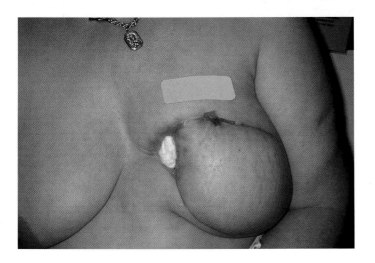

Figure 8.33
Wound packed with calcium alginate

Even larger wounds can be packed with this material, in either a sheet or rope configuration.

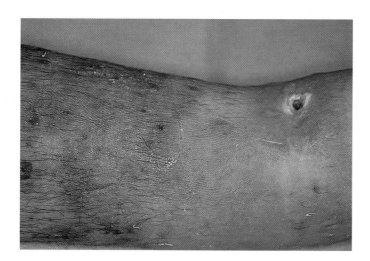

Figure 8.34a
Difficult wound management

This man had poliomyelitis as a child and multiple orthopedic procedures to his ankle. His clinical course was complicated by episodes of osteomyelitis. Eventually, he was left with a deep, non-healing ulcer on his ankle. This probably represents a sinus tract and there is considerable exudate. At the same time, the leg is affected by severe venous disease and edema.

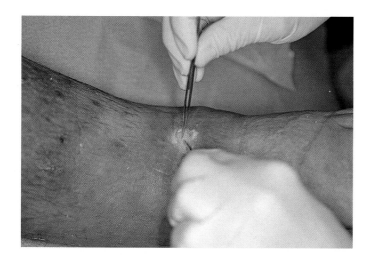

Figure 8.34b
Difficult wound management/Exudate control

The challenge in this case was to control the exudate and still apply compression bandages that would not have to be changed daily. It was decided to pack the sinus with calcium alginate and to create a window in the compression bandage that would allow daily wound dressing. Here, in this photograph, the wound is being gently packed with the calcium alginate material.

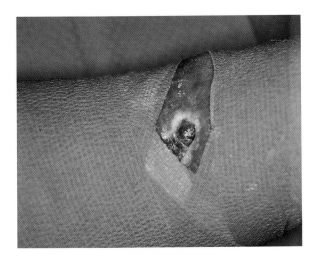

Figure 8.34c
Difficult wound management/Exudate control

After the elastic bandage was applied to the leg, a window was created right over the wound.

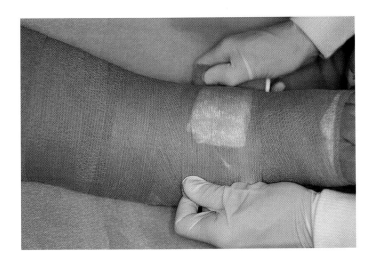

Figure 8.34d
Difficult wound management/Exudate control

A unit consisting of gauze and elastic bandage was placed immediately over the window and could provide additional absorbing capacity as well as re-establish compression. This unit could be changed daily or even more often by the patient or visiting nurse, while the leg compression would only be changed weekly.

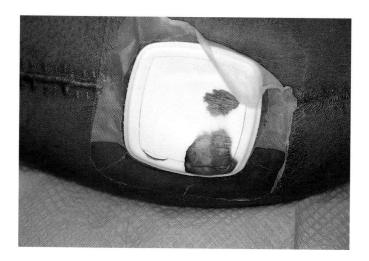

Figure 8.35a
Composite wound dressing

Situations arise when there is no ideal wound dressing available in the office. Then, one can combine different dressings to fit the need. This young paraplegic woman had wound dehiscence after a surgical procedure on her left hip. The defect was 5 cm deep and drained considerably. It was decided to pack the wound with calcium alginate and to provide additional absorption capacity with an overlying foam dressing. An island foam dressing was chosen because it would stay on better during repositioning of the patient and frequent transfers from bed to wheelchair. The photograph shows drainage in the foam island dressing, which indicates that it is time to change it.

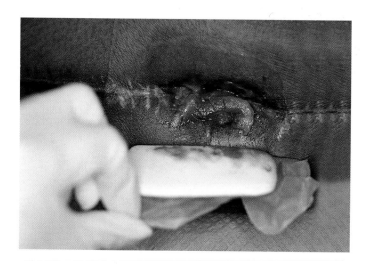

Figure 8.35b
Composite wound dressing/Removal

Upon removal of the foam dressing the calcium alginate rope packing material is visible and has become gelatinous. It can be removed easily.

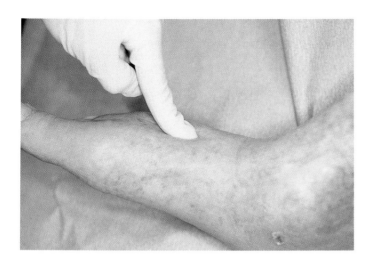

Figure 8.36
Pedal edema

The photograph shows pitting edema of the dorsum of the foot. Pedal edema can result from inadequate compression. It is important to apply compression bandages starting at the toes.

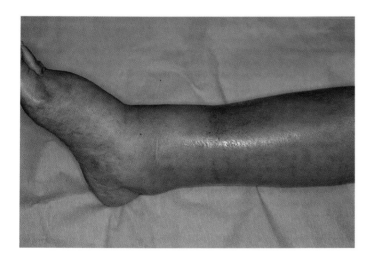

Figure 8.37
Leg edema

The entire leg became quite edematous when the patient failed to wear the elastic stockings that had been prescribed for the treatment of venous disease. Compliance with the use of stockings is a serious problem.

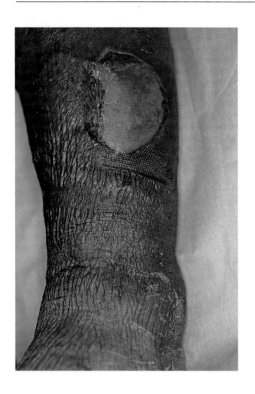

Figure 8.38
Edema and blistering

Blisters can develop in the setting of severe leg edema. Because such blisters can lead to chronic ulcers, it is important to establish compression therapy immediately. Another clinical consideration here would be streptococcal or staphylococcal infection, which can present as blisters.

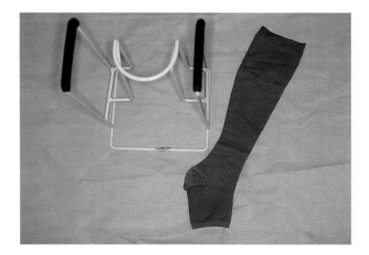

Figure 8.39a
Compression stockings

There are different types on the market and some are claimed to be easier to put on. Ironically, it is the people who need them the most who have difficulty with putting them on: the elderly, the obese, the patient with limited mobility. A "butler" device can facilitate the use of stockings, mainly for people with limited strength or ability to stretch the stocking over the foot.

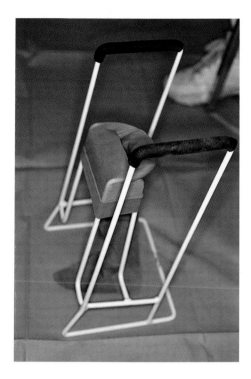

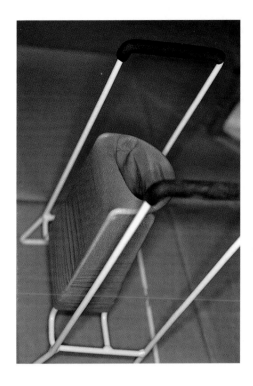

Figure 8.39b
Compression stocking/Use of butler

The patient holds the stocking inside the top semi-circular frame and pulls the top of the stocking over it, with the heel facing the back of the device.

Figure 8.39c
Compression stocking/Use of butler

One continues to slide the stocking down the semi-circular frame until it reaches the heel.

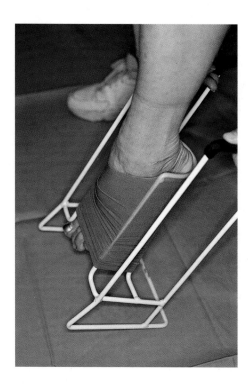

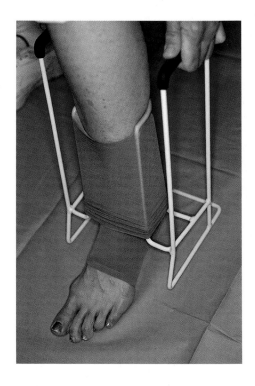

Figure 8.39d
Compression stocking/Use of butler

While sitting , the patient keeps inserting their foot in the stocking until it touches the floor.

Figure 8.39e
Compression stocking/Use of butler

By grasping the handles of the butler and pulling gently upward, one is able to slide the stocking up the leg.

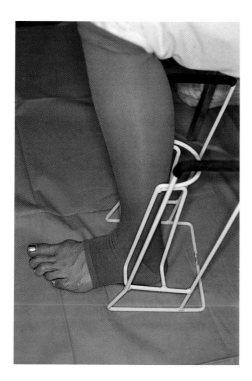

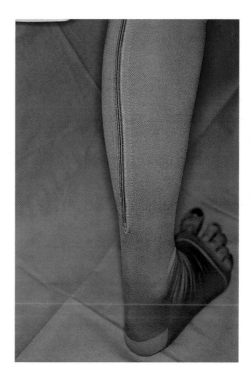

Figure 8.39f
Compression stocking/Use of butler

Once the process is mastered, it takes less strength and dexterity for patients to apply stockings using this device. It should be noted from this photograph that the stocking appears to be too short for this patient, so that less than the desired portion of the foot is being treated. Although many stockings can be bought over the counter, it is often necessary to obtain accurate measurements for best results.

Figure 8.40
Stockings with zippers

There have been other attempts to make stockings more "friendly". The incorporation of zippers in the stocking can facilitate their use. This still requires strength and dexterity to get the foot into the stocking and then to close the zipper on the back of the stocking.

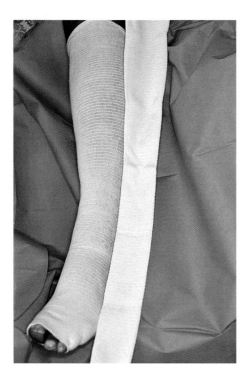

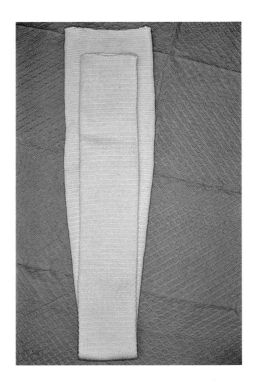

Figure 8.41a
Shaped support bandage

Shaped support bandages can be used as a primary compression bandage or for short-term use while a patient is healed and waiting for their stockings. Unlike regular tube gauze, this is specifically made smaller at the ankle and larger at the calf area to produce graduated compression.

Figure 8.41b
Shaped support bandage

These dressings come as one per package and the patient needs to be measured as directed at the ankle and calf, and for leg length, to prescribe the size that will give them the correct amount of pressure.

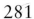

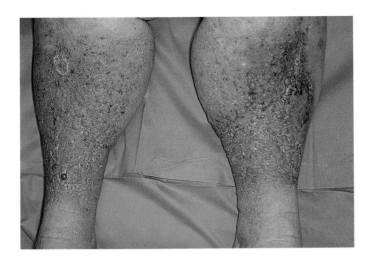

Figure 8.42a
Difficult-to-compress legs

There are patients in whom the
application of compression
bandages or stockings is either
difficult or impractical. This
particular patient with combined
venous and lymphatic disease is an
example. Such patients are
candidates for compression
pumps.

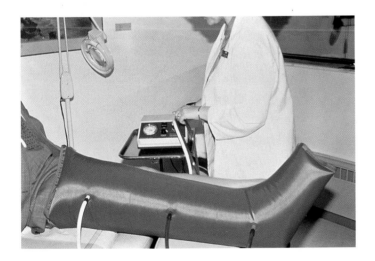

Figure 8.42b
Difficult-to-compress legs/Pump

These devices can be very helpful
in removing edema and managing
lymphedematous legs. It has also
been stated that they can help heal
wounds by removing edema.

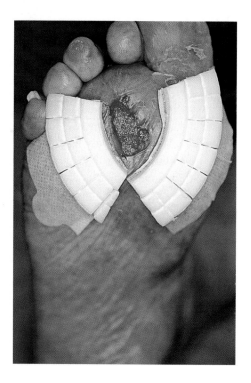

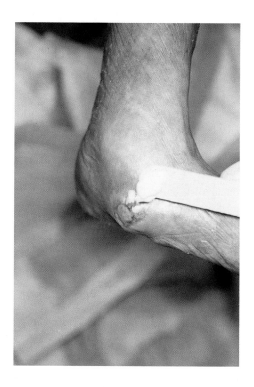

Figure 8.43
Ulcer protection

This woman confined to a wheelchair has had ulcerative lichen planus, which has required repeated intralesional injections of corticosteroids. This pressure relief foam dressing was trimmed of its hydrocolloid center to create two protective barriers around the wound. This helped protect the wound from trauma. One could also use other methods to protect the wound, such as a removable Scotchcast boot. The latter is rather often used in the UK for pressure ulcers or to protect the foot against trauma.

Figure 8.44a
Foot ulcer in rheumatoid arthritis

This elderly woman is confined to a wheelchair and is on systemic corticosteroids. This ulcer was difficult to heal and to keep healed. It would be another case where a Scotchcast boot would be helpful. In this case, the wound was managed with topical antibiotics and protective dressings. Here one sees the application of silver sulfadiazine.

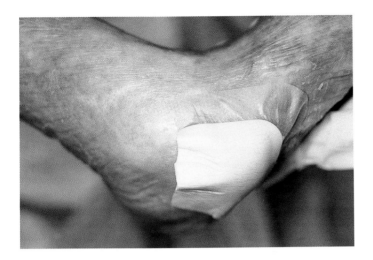

Figure 8.44b
Foot ulcer in rheumatoid arthritis

A foam island dressing was used to provide absorption of exudate and to act as a protective barrier. The dressing adheres well to difficult areas, such as this one, its border being a thin flexible film. At other times in this patient's clinical course, we have used wool padding to fill in the areas adjacent to the bony prominence where the ulcer is located. This allowed us to use compression bandages to control the edema.

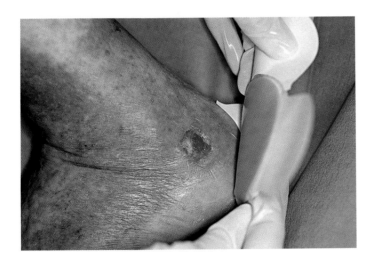

Figure 8.45a
Occlusion in difficult locations

At times, the location of the ulcer makes it very difficult to apply certain dressings. A dressing we have found to be helpful in these circumstances is a hydrocolloid dressing with paper tape "wings". Here it is being applied to this heel ulcer.

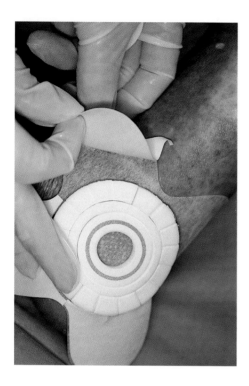

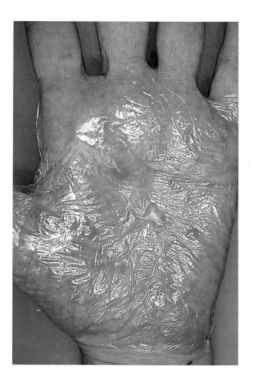

Figure 8.45b
Occlusion in difficult locations

The hydrocolloid portion is over the ulcer.
Rings of foam on the outside act as a
protective barrier. One can remove as many
of these rings as needed, based on the size of
the ulcer.

Figure 8.46
Film dressing for hand fissures

This patient had extremely painful fissures
occurring in the setting of hand dermatitis. A
film dressing was used to protect her hand
and relieve the intense pain. A skin adhesive
at the edges of the dressing in intact areas of
the skin ensured better and longer-lasting
adherence.

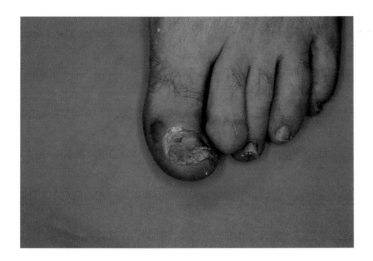

Figure 8.47a
Blister from pemphigus vulgaris

This life-threatening disorder is associated with antibodies to certain components of skin. It commonly causes oral ulcerations. Here a blister was present on the big toe. It was very painful and difficult to manage. This area would rub against the patient's shoe and needed a bandage system that would stay in place.

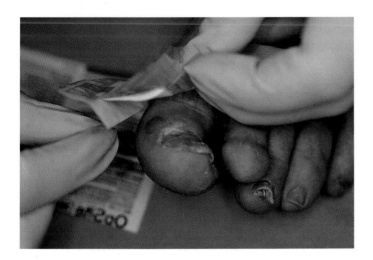

Figure 8.47b
Blister from pemphigus vulgaris/Dressing

A film dressing with an island of non-adherent material in the center turned out to be ideal. Here one can see the application, as the backing is removed from the island dressing.

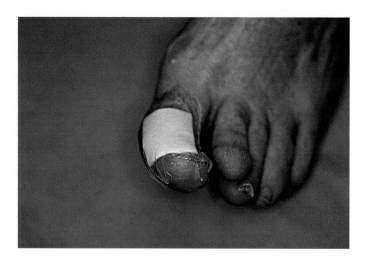

Figure 8.47c
Blister from pemphigus vulgaris/Dressing

The dressing provided a barrier between the blister and the shoe and adhered very well in this location. The patient was also able to shower without having to change the dressing.

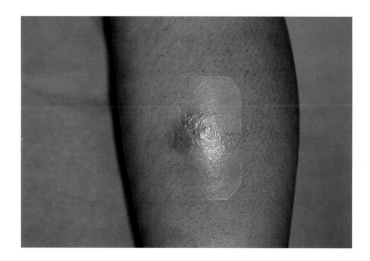

Figure 8.48a
Application of a film dressing

Films are very useful in wound management and, as observed here, can hardly be seen when applied to a wound or erosion. This is a very attractive feature. However, the trick is to apply films properly and without wrinkles, or else they become quite noticeable and also lose their protective barrier function.

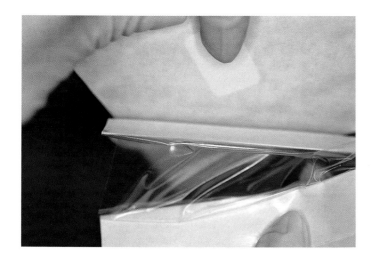

Figure 8.48b
Application of a film dressing

One must avoid self-adherence of the dressing when removing its backing. This backing is there to keep the dressing stable during application and is removed gradually during the application process. Here one sees that a portion of the film has become self-adherent. There are differences among different brands in how commonly this occurs and whether the film has the capacity to be unstuck.

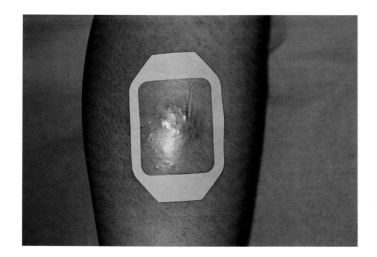

Figure 8.48c
Application of a film dressing

These dressings can be applied to the wound with the frame still present around them. The frame provides support during the application process and can be peeled off easily once the dressing is in place.

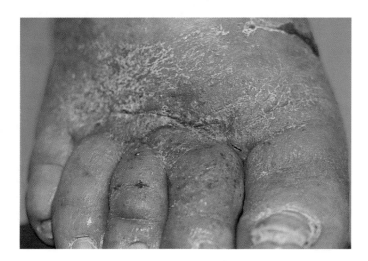

Figure 8.49a
Management of dermatitis

Wounds, especially those caused by venous disease, are frequently complicated by dermatitis. In our experience, topical antibiotics and emollients are the most common reasons for this problem. In treating this complication, we advice the use of films or hydrogels. The photograph shows a rather severe dermatitis on the dorsum of the foot and between the toes. Although the patient had onychomycosis, the scaling and dermatitis was not due to fungal infection.

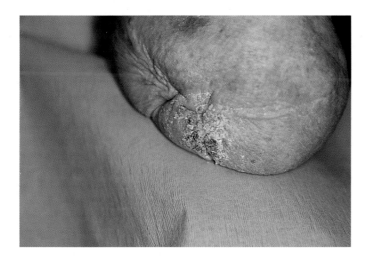

Figure 8.49b
Management of dermatitis

The dermatitic area over this stump was a rather serious problem because it prevented the use of the prosthetic. We also biopsied this scaly area to exclude the possibility of a squamous cell carcinoma, which could present in this way. This is another example where a hydrogel is helpful.

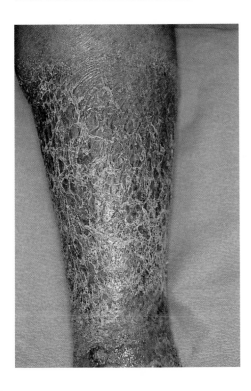

Figure 8.49c
Management of dermatitis

Here is yet another example where we would use a
hydrogel to control the severe dermatitis occurring in
the setting of venous insufficiency.

Selected bibliography

Bays HE, Pfeifer MA
Peripheral diabetic neuropathy. *Med Clin North Am* (1988) **72**:1439–1464.

Berry DP, Harding KG, Stanton MR, Jasani B, Ehrlich P
Human wound contraction: collagen organisation, fibroblasts, and myofibroblasts. *Plast Reconstr Surg* (1998) **102**:124–131.

Bizer LS, Ramos S, Weiss PR
A prospective randomized double blind study of perioperative antibiotic use in the grafting of ulcers of the lower extremity. *Surg Gynecol Obstet* (1992) **175**:113–114.

Black MM, Walkden VM
Basal cell carcinomatous changes on the lower leg: a possible association with chronic venous stasis. *Histopathology* (1983) **7**:219–227.

Blauvelt A, Falanga V
Idiopathic and L-tryptophan associated eosinophilic fasciitis before and after L-tryptophan contamination. *Arch Dermatol* (1991) **127**:1159–1166.

Boulton AJM
The diabetic foot. *Med Clin North Am* (1988) **72**:1513–1529.

Brodland DG, Staats BA, Peters MS
Factitial leg ulcers associated with an unusual sleep disorder. *Arch Dermatol* (1989) **125**:1115–1118.

Browse NL, Burnand KG
The cause of venous ulceration. *Lancet* (1982) **2**:243–245.

Browse NL, Gray L, Jarrett PEM, Morland M
Blood and vein-wall fibrinolytic activity in health and vascular disease. *Br Med J* (1977) **1**:478–481.

Bucalo B, Eaglstein WH, Falanga V
Inhibition of cell proliferation by chronic wound fluid. *Wound Rep Reg* (1993) **1**:181–186.

Burnand K, Clemenson G, Morland M, Jarrett PEM, Browse NL
Venous lipodermatosclerosis: treatment by fibrinolytic enhancement and elastic compression. *Br Med J* (1980) **280**:7–11.

Burnand K, Lea Thomas M, O'Donnell T, Browse NL
Relation between postphlebitic changes in the deep veins and results of surgical treatment of venous ulcers. *Lancet* (1976) **i**:936–938.

Burnand KG, O'Donnell TF, Lea Thomas M, Browse NL
The relative importance of incompetent communicating veins in the production of varicose veins and venous ulcers. *Surgery* (1977) **82**:9–14.

Callam MJ, Harper DR, Dale JJ, Ruckley CV
Chronic ulcer of the leg: clinical history. *Br Med J* (1987) **294**:1389–1391.

Callam MJ, Harper DR, Dale JJ, Ruckley CV
A controlled trial of weekly ultrasound therapy in chronic leg ulceration. *Lancet* (1987) **ii**:204–206.

Claudy AL, Mirshahi M, Soria C, Soria J
Detection of undegraded fibrin and tumor necrosis factor-alpha in venous leg ulcers. *J Am Acad Dermatol* (1991) **25**:623–627.

Coleridge Smith PD
The microcirculation in venous hypertension. *Cardiovasc Res* (1996) **32**:769–795.

Coleridge Smith P, Sarin Sanjeev, Hasty J, Scurr JH
Sequential gradient pneumatic compression enhances venous ulcer healing: a randomized trial. *Surgery* (1990) **108**:871–875.

Colgan M-P, Dormandy JA, Jones PW, Schraibman IG, Shanik DG, Young RAL
Oxpentifylline treatment of venous ulcers of the leg. *Br Med J* (1990) **300**:972–975.

Cutting KF, Harding KG
Criteria for identifying wound infection. *J Wound Care* (1994) **3**:198–201.

Dahn MS
The role of growth factors in wound management of diabetic foot ulcers. *Fed Pract* (1998) July:14–19.

De Ceulaer K, Khamashta MA, Harris EN, Serjeant GR, Hughes GRV
Antiphospholipid antibodies in homozygous sickle cell disease. *Ann Rheum Dis* (1992) **51**:671–672.

Dvorak HF
Tumors: wounds that do not heal. *N Engl J Med* (1986) **315**:1650–1659.

Eaglstein WH, Davis SC, Mehle AI, Mertz PM
Optimal use of an occlusive dressing to enhance healing: effect of delayed application and early removal on wound healing. *Arch Dermatol* (1988) **124**:392–395.

Elgart G, Stover P, Larson K et al
Treatment of pyoderma gangrenosum with cyclosporine: results in seven patients. *J Am Acad Dermatol* (1991) **24**:83–86.

English MP, Smith RJ, Harman RRM
The fungal flora of ulcerated legs. *Br J Dermatol* (1971) **84**:567–582.

Falanga V
Chronic wounds: pathophysiologic and experimental considerations. *J Invest Dermatol* (1993) **100**:721–725.

Falanga V
Iodine-containing pharmaceuticals: a reappraisal. In: *Proceedings of the 6th European Conference on Advances in Wound Management* (Macmillan Magazines Ltd: London, 1997) 191–194.

Falanga V
Venous ulceration. In: Krasner D, Kane D, eds. *Chronic Wound Care: A Clinical Source Book for Health Care Professionals*. (Health Management Publications, Inc., 1997) 165–171.

Falanga V, Carson P, Greenberg A, Hasan A, Nichols E, McPherson J
Topically applied tPA for the treatment of venous ulcers. *Dermatol Surg* (1996) **22**:643–644.

Falanga V, Eaglstein WH
The trap hypothesis of venous ulceration. *Lancet* (1993) **341**:1006–1008.

Falanga V, Eaglstein WH
Leg and Foot Ulcers: A Clinician's Guide (Martin Dunitz: London, 1995) 154–155.

Falanga V, Grinnell F, Gilchrest B, Maddox YT, Moshell A
Experimental approaches to chronic wounds. *Wound Rep Reg* (1995) **3**:132–140.

Falanga V, Kruskal JB, Franks JJ
Fibrin and fibrinogen-related antigens in patients with venous disease and venous ulceration. *Arch Dermatol* (1991) **127**:75–78.

Falanga V, Kirsner RS, Eaglstein WH, Katz MH, Kerdel FA
Stanozolol in treatment of leg ulcers due to cryofibrinogenemia. *Lancet* (1991) **338**:347–348.

Falanga V, Margolis D, Alvarez O et al
Healing of venous ulcers and lack of clinical rejection with an allogeneic cultured human skin equivalent. *Arch Dermatol* (1998) **134**:293–300.

Falanga V, Moosa HH, Nemeth AJ, Alstadt SP, Eaglstein WH
Dermal pericapillary fibrin in venous ulceration. *Arch Dermatol* (1987) **123**: 620–623.

Falstie-Jensen N, Spaun E, Brochner-Mortensen J, Falstie-Jensen S
The influence of epidermal thickness on transcutaneous oxygen pressure measurements in normal persons. *Scand J Clin Lab Invest* (1988) **48**:519–523.

Fine MJ, Kapoor W, Falanga V
Cholesterol crystal embolization: a review of 22l cases in the English literature. *Angiology* (1987) **38**:769–784.

Fletcher A, Cullum N, Sheldon TA
A systematic review of compression treatment for venous leg ulcers. *Br Med J* (1997) **315**:576–580.

Fraki JE, Peltonen L, Hopsu-Havu VK
Allergy to various components of topical preparations in stasis dermatitis and leg ulcer. *Contact Dermatitis* (1979) **5**:97–100.

Gentzkow GD, Iwasaki SD, Hershon KS et al
Use of dermagraft, a cultured human dermis, to treat diabetic foot ulcers. *Diabetes Care* (1996) **19**:350–354.

Gilchrist B, Reed C
The bacteriology of chronic venous ulcers treated with occlusive hydrocolloid dressings. *Br J Dermatol* (1989) **121**:337–344.

Gilman TH
Parameter for measurement of wound closure. *Wounds* (1990) **3**:95–101.

Goldman MP, Weiss RA, Bergan JJ
Diagnosis and treatment of varicose veins: a review. *J Am Acad Dermatol* (1994) **31**:393–413.

Gowland Hopkins NF, Jamieson CW
Antibiotic concentration in the exudate of venous ulcers: the prediction of healing rate. *Br J Surg* (1983) **70**:532–534.

Gowland Hopkins NF, Spinks TJ, Rhodes CG, Ranicar ASO, Jamieson CW
Positron emission tomography in venous ulceration and liposclerosis: study of regional tissue function. *Br Med J* (1983) **286**:333–336.

Greenberg AS, Hasan T, Montalvo BM, Falabella A, Falanga V
Acute lipodermatosclerosis is associated with venous insufficiency. *J Am Acad Dermatol* (1996) **35**:566–568.

Grob JJ, San Marco M, Aillaud MF et al
Unfading acral microlivedo. A discrete marker of thrombotic skin disease associated with antiphospholipid antibody syndrome. *J Am Acad Dermatol* (1991) **24**:53–58.

Harding KG
Wound healing: putting theory into clinical practice. *Wounds* (1990) **2**:21–32.

Harris B, Eaglstein WH, Falanga V
Basal cell carcinoma arising in venous ulcers and mimicking granulation tissue. *J Dermatol Surg Oncol* (1993) **19**:150–152.

Harrison PV
Split-skin grafting of varicose leg ulcers – a survey and the importance of assessment of risk factors in predicting outcome from the procedure. *Clin Exp Dermatol* (1988) **13**:4–6.

Hasan A, Murata H, Falabella A et al
Dermal fibroblasts from venous ulcers are unresponsive to the action of transforming growth factor-β 1. *J Dermatol Sci* (1997) **16**:59–66.

Helfman T, Ovington L, Falanga V
Occlusive dressings and wound healing. *Clin Dermatol* (1994) **12**:121–127.

Hendricks WM, Swallow RT
Management of stasis leg ulcers with Unna's boots versus elastic support stockings. *J Am Acad Dermatol* (1985) **12**:90–98.

Higley HR, Ksander GA, Gerhardt CO, Falanga V
Extravasation of macromolecules and possible trapping of TGF-beta in venous ulceration. *Br J Dermatol* (1995) **132**:79–85.

Hook EW, Hooton TM, Horton CA, Coyle MB, Ramsey PG, Turck M
Microbiologic evaluation of cutaneous cellulitis in adults. *Arch Intern Med* (1986) **146**:295–297.

Hunt TK, Ehrlich HP, Garcia JA, Englebert Dunphy J
Effect of vitamin A on reversing the inhibitory effect of cortisone on healing of open wounds in animals and man. *Ann Surg* (1969) **170**:633–641.

Jian Wen G, Harding KG
Enhancement of wound tissue expansion and angiogenesis by matrix-embedded fibroblast (Dermagraft), a role of hepatocyte growth factor/scatter factor. *Plast Reconstr Surg* (1998) **2**:203–210.

Johnson RB, Lazarus GS
Pulse therapy. Therapeutic efficacy in the treatment of pyoderma gangrenosum. *Arch Dermatol* (1982) **118**:76–84.

Katz MH, Alvarez AF, Kirsner RS, Eaglstein WH, Falanga V
Human wound fluid from acute wounds stimulates fibroblast and endothelial cell growth. *J Am Acad Dermatol* (1991) **25**:1054–1058.

Kirsner RS, Falanga V, Eaglstein WH
The biology of skin grafts: skin grafts as pharmacologic agents. *Arch Dermatol* (1993) **129**:481–483.

Kirsner RS, Pardes JB, Eaglstein WH, Falanga V
The clinical spectrum of lipodermatosclerosis. *J Am Acad Dermatol* (1993) **28**:623–627.

Klein KL, Pittelkow MR
Tissue plasminogen activator for treatment of livedoid vasculitis. *Mayo Clin Proc* (1992) **67**:923–933.

Lawrence TW
Physiology of the acute wound. In: Granick MS, Long CD, Ramasastry SS, eds. *Clinics in Plastic Surgery. Wound Healing: State of the Art.* (WB Saunders Co.: Philadelphia, 1998) 321–340.

Lees T, Singh S, Beard J, Spencer P, Rigby C
Prospective audit of surgery for varicose veins. *Br J Surg* (1997) **84**:44–46.

Lewis CE, Antoine J, Mueller C, Talbot WA, Swaroop R, Sterling Edwards W
Elastic compression in the prevention of venous stasis. A critical reevaluation. *Am J Surg* (1976) **132**:739–743.

Lofgren KA, Lauvstad WA, Bonnemaison MF
Surgical treatment of large stasis ulcer: review of 129 cases. *Mayo Clin Proc* (1965) **40**:560–563.

LoGerfo FW, Coffman JD
Vascular and microvascular disease of the foot in diabetes. *N Engl J Med* (1984) **311**:1615–1619.

Marks J, Harding KG, Hughes LE, Ribeiro CD
Pilonidal sinus excision – healing by open granulation. *Br J Surg* (1985) **72**:637–640.

Marks J, Hughes LE, Harding KG, Campbell H, Ribeiro CD
Prediction of healing time as an aid to the management of open granulating wounds. *World J Surg* (1983) **7**:641–645.

McEnroe CS, O'Donnell TF, Mackey WC
Correlation of clinical findings with venous hemodynamics in 86 patients with chronic venous insufficiency. *Am J Surg* (1988) **156**:148–152.

Mitchell Sams W
Livedo vasculitis. Therapy with pentoxifylline. *Arch Dermatol* (1988) **124**:684–687.

Moore K, Ruge F, Harding KG
T lymphocytes and the lack of activated macrophages in wound margin biopsies from chronic leg ulcers. *Br J Dermatol* (1997) **137**:188–194.

Moore K, Thomas A, Harding KG
Iodine released from the wound dressing iodosorb modulates the secretion of cytokines by human macrophages responding to bacterial lipopolysaccharide. *Int J Biochemistry and Cell Biol* (1997) **29**:163–171.

Myers MB, Rightor M, Cherry GW
Relationship between oedema and the healing rate of stasis ulcers of the leg. *Am J Surg* (1972) **124**:66–68.

Nelson EA
Compression bandaging in the treatment of venous leg ulcers. *J Wound Care* (1996) **5**:415–418.

Nemeth AJ, Eaglstein WH, Falanga V
Clinical parameters and transcutaneous oxygen measurements for the prognosis of venous ulcers. *J Am Acad Dermatol* (1989) **20**:186–190.

Newman LG, Waller J, Palestro CJ et al
Unsuspected osteomyelitis in diabetic foot ulcers. *JAMA* (1991) **266**:1246–1251.

Nwomeh BC, Yager DR, Cohen IK
Physiology of the chronic wound. In: Granick MS, Long CD, Ramasastry SS, eds. *Clinics in Plastic Surgery. Wound Healing: State of the Art* (WB Saunders Co.: Philadelphia, 1998) 341–356.

O'Neill ID, Hopkinson I, Thomas DW, Harding KG, Shepherd JP
Pathogenesis of hypertrophic and keloid scarring. *Int J Oral Maxillofac Surg* (1994) **23**:232–236.

Ormiston MC, Seymour MTJ, Venn GE, Fox JA
Controlled trial of iodosorb in chronic venous ulcers. *Br Med J* (1985) **291**:308–310.

Partsch H
Compression therapy of the legs. A review. *J Dermatol Surg Oncol* (1991) **17**:799–805.

Phillips T
New skin for old. Developments in biological skin substitutes. *Arch Dermatol* (1998) **134**:344–349

Phillips TJ, Kehinde O, Green H, Gilchrest BA
Treatment of skin ulcers with cultured epidermal allografts. *J Am Acad Dermatol* (1989) **21**:191–199.

Phillips TJ, Salman SM, Rogers GS
Nonhealing leg ulcers: a manifestation of basal cell carcinoma. *J Am Acad Dermatol* (1991) **25**:47–49.

Phillips T, Stanton B, Provan A, Lew R
A study of the impact of leg ulcers on quality of life: financial, social, and psychological implications. *J Am Acad Dermatol* (1993) **19**:764–771.

Porter JM, Cutler BS, Lee BY et al
Pentoxifylline efficacy in the treatment of intermittent claudication: multicenter controlled double-blind trial with objective assessment of chronic occlusive arterial disease of patients. *Am Heart J* (1982) **104**:66–72.

Porter JM, Moneta GL
An international consensus committee on chronic venous disease. Reporting standards in venous disease: an update. *J Vasc Surg* (1995) **21**:635–645.

Prasad A, Ali-Khan A, Mortimer PS
Leg ulcers and oedema: a study exploring the prevalence, aetiology, and possible significance of oedema in venous ulcers. *Phlebology* (1990) **5**:181–187.

Rademaker M, Lowe DG, Munro DD
Erythema induratum (Bazin's disease). *J Am Acad Dermatol* (1989) **21**:740–745.

Ram Zvi, Sadeh M, Walden R, Adar R
Vascular insufficiency quantitatively aggravates diabetic neuropathy. *Arch Neurol* (1991) **48**:1239–1242.

Robson MC
Exogenous growth factor application effect on human wound healing. *Prog Dermatol* (1996) **30**:1–7.

Ruckley CV, Prescott RJ
Treatment of chronic leg ulcers. *Lancet* (1994) **344**:1512–1513.

Ruckley CV
Does venous reflux matter? *Lancet* (1993) **341**:411–412.

Sarin S, Cheatle TR, Coleridge Smith PD, Scurr JH
Disease mechanisms in venous ulceration. *Br J Hosp Med* (1991) **45**:303–305.

Scheffler A, Rieger H
A comparative analysis of transcutaneous oxymetry (tcPO$_2$) during oxygen inhalation and leg dependency in severe peripheral arterial occlusive disease. *J Vasc Surg* (1992) **16**:218–224.

Serjeant GR
Leg ulceration in sickle cell anemia. *Arch Intern Med* (1974) **133**:690–694.

Sigel B, Edelstein AL, Savitch L, Hasty JH, Robert Felix W
Type of compression for reducing venous stasis. A study of lower extremities during inactive recumbency. *Arch Surg* (1975) **110**:171–175.

Sindrup JH, Groth S, Avnstorp C, Tonnesen KH, Kristensen JK
Coexistence of obstructive arterial disease and chronic venous stasis in leg ulcer patients. *Clin Exp Dermatol* (1987) **12**:410–412.

Skene AI, Smith JM, Dore CJ, Charlett A, Lewis JD
Venous leg ulcers: a prognostic index to predict time to healing. *Br Med J* (1992) **305**:1119–1121.

Smiell JM
Clinical safety of becaplermin (rhPDGF-BB) gel. Becaplermin Studies Group. *Am J Surg* (1998) **176**: 68S-73S.

Smith RJ, English MP, Warin RP
The pathogenic status of yeasts infecting ulcerated legs. *Br J Dermatol* (1974) **91**:697–699.

Stacey MC, Burnand KG, Layer GT, Pattison M
Transcutaneous oxygen tensions in assessing the treatment of healed venous ulcers. *Br J Surg* (1990) **77**:1050–1054.

Steed DL, Donohoe D, Webster MW, Lindsley L
Effect of extensive debridement and treatment on the healing of diabetic foot ulcers. Diabetic Ulcer Study Group. *J Am Coll Surg* (1996) **183**:61–64.

Steed DL, Goslen JB, Holloway GA, Malone JM, Bunt TJ, Webster MW
Randomized prospective double-blind trial in healing chronic diabetic foot ulcers. CT-102 activated platelet supernatant, topical versus placebo. *Diabetes Care* (1992) **15**:1598–1604.

Steed DL, the Diabetic Ulcer Study Group
Clinical evaluation of recombinant human platelet-derived growth factor for the treatment of lower extremity diabetic ulcers. *J Vasc Surg* (1995) **21**: 71–81.

The Alexander House Group
Consensus paper on venous leg ulcers. *Phlebology* (1992) **7**:48–58.

Thomas DW, Harding KG, Shepherd JP
Cutaneous wound healing: a current perspective. *Int J Oral Maxillofac Surg* (1995) **53**:442–447.

Van de Scheur M, Falanga V
Pericapillary fibrin cuffs in venous disease. A reappraisal. *Dermatol Surg* (1997) **23**:955–959.

Vanscheidt W, Laaff H, Weiss JM, Schopf E
Immunohistochemical investigation of dermal capillaries in chronic venous insufficiency. *Acta Derm Venereol (Stockh)* (1991) **71**:17–19.

Wieman TJ, Griffiths GD, Polk HC
Management of diabetic midfoot ulcers. *Ann Surg* (1992) **215**:627–632.

Wieman TJ, Smiell JM, Su Y
Efficacy and safety of a topical gel formulation of recombinant human platelet-derived growth factor-BB (becaplermin) in patients with chronic neuropathic diabetic ulcers. A phase III randomized placebo-controlled double-blind study. *Diabetes Care* (1998) **21**:822–827.

Yao ST, Hobbs JT, Irvine WT
Ankle systolic pressure measurements in arterial disease affecting the lower extremities. *Br J Surg* (1969) **56**:676–679.

Wertheim D, Melhuish J, Wiliams R, Harding KG
Measurement of forces associated with compression therapy. *Med Biol Eng Comput* (1999) **37**:31–34.

Whiston RJ, Hallett MB, Davies EV, Harding KG, Lane IF
Inappropriate neutrophil activation in venous disease. *Br J Surg* (1994) **81**:695–698.

Woods GL, Washington JA
Mycobacteria other than *Mycobacterium tuberculosis*: review of microbiologic and clinical aspects. *Rev Infect Dis* (1987) **9**:275–294.

Index